MW00837599

Neuropathology and Neuroradiology
A Review

Aug 27, 2001

2004 -- renewed.

renewed.

Dec. 31, 2005.

Oct 28 2005

Fax. (219) 756 - 5540

NEUROPATHOLOGY AND NEURORADIOLOGY: A REVIEW

Jonathan Stuart Citow, M.D.

Clinical Assistant Professor
Department of Neurosurgery
University of Chicago Medical Center
Chicago, Illinois

Robert L. Wollmann, M.D., Ph.D.

Professor
Departments of Pathology and Neurology
University of Chicago Medical Center
Chicago, Illinois

Robert L. Macdonald, M.D., Ph.D.

Associate Professor
Department of Neurosurgery
University of Chicago Medical Center
Chicago, Illinois

Foreword by Bryce Weir, O.C., M.D.

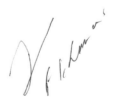

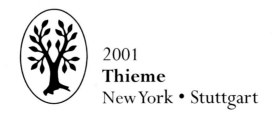

2001
Thieme
New York • Stuttgart

Table of Contents

Foreword

The best books are those which take from the reader the least amount of time and money in return for the most information. Dr. Citow and colleagues have done yeoman work in distilling the vast corpus of clinical neuroscience into this concise, yet readable book. The illustrations portray essential information. Young neurosurgeons preparing for the hurdles for professional examinations will find this to be a most valuable aid. I suspect that those who use it and become familiar with its contents will continue to browse through it as the years go by to refresh their memories. All those involved in the care of patients with neurological diseases will read this work to their advantage. It is remarkable that Dr. Citow had the ability to write this book while still in his residency. Future residents will have reason to be grateful for his industry.

Bryce Weir, O.C., M.D.
Maurice Goldblatt Professor of Surgery and Neurosurgery
The University of Chicago
Chicago, Illinois

Preface

The fields of neuropathology and neuroradiology are advancing daily. New immuno-histochemical and other staining methods help us to more accurately categorize pathologic processes. New radiologic studies (i.e., PET scan, SPECT scan, CT angiography) are adding invaluable information that enhances our ability to manage difficult patients. We are now able to be more certain of our diagnoses and lesion localization than ever before, yet these fields remain as much an art as a science. There are always bizarre exceptions that challenge the most renowned experts. In this book, I have attempted to summarize most of the important facts about the more common neurological diseases and include classical pathology slides and radiographic images to help the students of these disciplines become comfortable with their diagnoses.

Jonathan Stuart Citow, M.D.

References

Diagnostic Neuroradiology. Osborne AG. St. Louis, MO: Mosby, 1994.

Neuroradiology, 3rd Edition. Ramsey RG. Philadelphia, PA: W.B. Saunders, Co., 1994.

Principles and Practice of Neuropathology. Nelson JS, Parisi JE, Schochet SS (Eds.). St Louis, MO: Mosby, 1993.

Principles of Neurology, 5th Edition. Adams RD, Victor M. New York: McGraw Hill, 1993.

Neurological Surgery, 4th Edition. Youmans JR (Ed.). Philadelphia, PA: W.B. Saunders, Inc., 1994.

Handbook of Neurosurgery, 3rd Edition. Greenberg MS. Lakeland, FL: Greenberg Graphics, Co., 1996.

Core Text of Neuroanatomy, 4th Edition. Carpenter MB. Baltimore, MD: Williams & Wilkins, 1991.

Atlas of Human Anatomy, 7th Edition. Netter FH. Summit, NJ: CIBA-Geigy, 1994.

Clinically Oriented Anatomy, 3rd Edition. Moore KL. Baltimore, MD: Williams & Wilkins, 1992.

Acknowledgments

I wish to thank Robert Wollmann for all of his help in obtaining the pathology slides and for imparting a very small percentage of his tremendous pathology knowledge to me and my fellow physicians at the University of Chicago. I wish to thank Rao Nadimpalli for lending me some of his rare yet classic X-rays. I wish to thank Loch Macdonald for all of his editing help and neurosurgical teachings. I wish to thank Lydia Johns for all of her help in developing the images. I wish to thank Bryce Weir for keeping me focused in my training. Finally, I wish to thank my partners Jeffery Karasick and Sheldon Lazar for helping me find the time to complete this project.

Jonathan Stuart Citow, M.D.

I. GENERAL NEUROPATHOLOGY

A. Neural stains—haematoxylin and eosin (H & E) are used for general pathologic examination. The Nissl stain is used to demonstrate neuron cell bodies (it binds nucleic acid). The silver stain demonstrates cell processes such as axions and dendrites. Lipofuscin accumulates in the central nervous system (CNS) neurons with aging. Neuromelanin accumulates in neurons (especially the substantia nigra (SN) and locus ceruleus) and is a catecholamine waste product (it is not made by tyrosinase). True melanin is made by **tyrosinase** and is located in the leptomeningeal melanocytes of the **ventral medulla and cervical cord**. These cells form the primary CNS melanomas.

B. Edema (increased brain water)

   1. Vasogenic edema—due to increased **blood-brain barrier (BBB) permeability** to proteins and macromolecules. It is caused by vessel damage, inflammation, and neovascularity. It is the most common type of edema, is **extracellular**, and effects the white matter more than the gray matter. **Steroids** are of value in decreasing this type of edema.

   2. Cytotoxic edema—caused by an **impaired Na^+/K^+ pump** related to decreased ATP delivery during hypoxia and ischemia. Water and electrolytes accumulate in the cell but not plasma proteins. It is **intracellular**, effects both the gray and white matter, and is not associated with CT or MRI enhancement because of the intact BBB. Steroids do not help decrease the edema.

   3. Interstitial edema—the transependymal shift of fluid caused by cerebral spinal fluid (CSF) accumulation (hydrocephalus) and is extracellular.

C. Lethal neuronal injury—characterized by ischemic necrosis. The cytoplasm that was slightly basophilic becomes eosinophilic (red is dead), and the nucleus becomes shrunken and dark. Changes can be seen within 6 hours. Ferrugination occurs when dead neurons become encrusted with Fe^{++} and Ca^{++} salts.

D. Progressive or reversible neuronal injury is characterized by:

1. Central chromatolysis—occurs after an injury to an axon near the cell body. The Nissl substance disappears, the nucleus becomes eccentric, and the cell body enlarges. It is seen with anterior nerve root compression and Guillain-Barré syndrome in the anterior horn cells. The cells may progress to death or recover.

2. Neurofibrillary degeneration—argyrophillic linear densities accumulate in the cell bodies and processes. They can be detected on silver stain. The neurofibrils are made of microtubules (tubulin), neurofilaments, and microfilaments (actin). The densities are much more numerous with Alzheimer's disease, postencephalitic Parkinson's disease, progressive supranuclear palsy, and aluminum toxicity.

3. Neuronal storage of lipids or carbohydrates—the cell body enlarges, the nucleus becomes eccentric, and the cytoplasm becomes foamy.

4. Inclusion bodies

   (a) Viral
       (i) **Intranuclear**—Herpes simplex virus type I (Cowdry type A, eosinophilic, in neurons, astrocytes, and oligodendrocytes, seen early in the disease), cytomegalovirus (CMV), and measles subacute sclerosing pan-encephalitis (SSPE).
       (ii) **Intracytoplasmic**—Rabies (Negri bodies), SSPE, and CMV.
   (b) Degenerative/metabolic (**all intracytoplasmic**)—Pick bodies (in Pick's disease, round, stains with silver), Lewy bodies (in Parkinson's disease, has a halo), Lafora's bodies (in Lafora's disease, PAS positive, basophilic, has a dense core), Hirano bodies (eosinophilic, most in hippocampus, seen in the elderly and increased with Alzheimer's disease), and Bunina bodies (eosinophilic, increased with amyotropiz lateral sclerosis [ALS]).

5. Marinesco bodies are seen in normal brains, are eosinophilic, and are located in the melanin cells of the brain stem.

E. Neuronal atrophy—occurs with degenerative diseases and has been postulated to be due to either excitatory amino acids, subcellular injuries by free radicals, or gene-directed apoptosis. Neuronal atrophy is associated with proliferation of astrocytes and microglia.

F. Hamartoma—disorganized cells in the proper location for that cell type.

G. Choristoma—correctly organized cells in the wrong location.

H. Brain herniation changes—**Kernohan's notch** (the contralateral cerebral peduncle is compressed against the incisura with ipsilateral weakness producing a false localizing sign), posterior cerebral artery (PCA) stroke, **Duret's hemorrhages** of the midbrain and pons (by arteriole stretching), cranial nerve (CN) III nerve palsy, and hydrocephalus (by compression of the cerebral aqueduct).

II. GLIAL CELL RESPONSE TO INJURY

A. Astrocytes—either protoplasmic (mainly in the gray matter) or fibrillary (mainly in the white matter). Glial fibrillary acidic protein (GFAP) is the main component of astrocytic **intermediate filaments**.

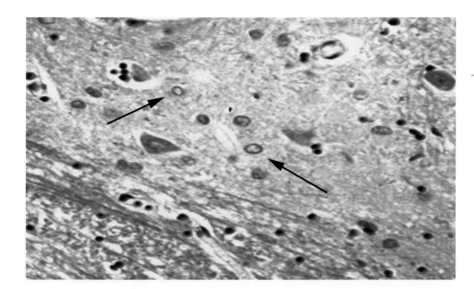

Figure 1   Alzheimer type 2 astrocytes (H and E); large vesicular nuclei with little cytoplasm (arrows).

B. Astrocytic reaction to injury

1. Secondary (reactive) astrocytosis—occurs after strokes, degenerative diseases, etc. There rarely are mitotic figures unless there is neoplastic disease. Gemistocytic astrocytes are large reactive astrocytes with eccentric nuclei. Fibrillary astrocytes appear later, have smaller cell bodies, and more fibers. **Rosenthal fibers** are eosinophilic masses in the astrocytic processes and are increased with **Alexander's disease**, **pilocytic astrocytomas**, and **astrocytosis**.

2. Primary astrocytosis—the proliferation of astrocytes after astrocytic disease such as hepatic encephalopathy with **Alzheimer II astrocytes** (large nuclei, gray, glycogen inclusions) (**Fig. 1**).

C. Microglia—macrophages from outside the CNS. With mild injury, there may be **rod cells** with cigar-shaped nuclei.

D. Oligodendrocytes—proliferate around multiple sclerosis (MS) plaques and are increased in size with bizarre shapes around the periphery in progressive multifocal leukoencephalopathy (PML).

E. Ependymal cells—do not proliferate with injury, but when damaged are replaced by subependymal astrocytes.

III. NERVOUS SYSTEM DEVELOPMENT

A. Three percent of newborns have major structural abnormalities, and most involve the CNS.

B. The brain and spinal cord are formed from neuroectoderm at 3 to 8 weeks. **Primary neurulation** occurs at 3 to 4 weeks with formation of the neural plate, neural groove, and neural folds. The **primitive streak** forms at postovulatory day 13. The **notochord** forms at day 17 and induces the primitive streak to form the **neural plate** that later develops the **neural groove** and **neural folds**. The neural folds fuse at 22 days to form the neural tube, with the proximal two-thirds forming the brain and the distal one-third forming the spinal cord. It closes like a zipper starting at the **hindbrain** with the **anterior neuropore closing first** at 24 days (forming the **lamina terminalis**) and the posterior end closing second (to L1/2) at 26 days. A problem at this stage causes neural tube defects and Chiari malformations.

C. **Disjunction**—the separation of ectoderm from neuroectoderm after the neural tube forms. The mesenchyme in between the two layers forms dura, neural arches, and paraspinal muscles. If disjunction occurs too early, the mesenchyme can enter the neural tube and form lipomas and lipomyelomeningoceles. Focal failure of disjunction causes an epithelial-lined dermal sinus tract. Larger failure of disjunction causes a myelocele or a myelomeningocele.

D. **Secondary neurulation**—occurs at 4 to 5 weeks as the mesoderm forms the dura, skull, vertebrae, and distal spine. Defects of secondary neurulation cause spinal dysraphism below L1/2.

E. Ventral induction—occurs at 5 to 10 weeks as the primary vesicles form from the neural tube (see following). Abnormalities at this stage cause holoprosencephaly, septo-optic dysplasia, and Dandy-Walker malformation. **Induction** is the growing brain's influence on the overlying mesoderm causing it to grow.

F. Neuronal proliferation and differentiation—occur at 2 to 4 months. A problem at this stage causes vascular malformations and neurocutaneous syndromes.

G. Cellular migration—occurs at 2 to 5 months with migration of cells from the deeper layers to more superficial layers, except for the outer cortical layer. A problem at this stage causes callosal agenesis, schizencephaly, and heterotopias.

H. Neuronal organization and myelination—occur from 5 months to the postnatal period as the synapses form. Myelination begins in the fifth fetal month and proceeds caudad to cephalad, dorsal to ventral, central to peripheral, and sensory before motor. Most is completed by 2 years. At birth the cortex/white matter signals on MRI are reversed because of the paucity of myelination and increased water content of the cortex compared with the white matter.

I. At 4 to 5 weeks, the prosencephalon, mesencephalon, and rhombencephalon form. The **prosencephalon** then divides into (1) the **telencephalon** that forms the hemispheres, **caudate**, **putamen**, fornices, **anterior commissure**, corpus callosum, and hippocampus; and (2) the **diencephalon** that forms the thalamus, **globus pallidus (GP)**, posterior hypophysis, **infundibulum**, **optic nerve**, **retina**, **posterior commissure**, and the habenular commissure. The **mesencephalon** forms the midbrain. The **rhombencephalon** divides into (1) the **metencephalon** that forms the pons and **cerebellum**, and (2) the **myelencephalon** that forms the medulla.

J. **Germinal matrix**—forms at 7 weeks and produces neurons and glia. At 30 weeks, the germinal matrix involutes (although some clusters exist until 39 weeks).

K. Commissures—form at 8 to 17 weeks. The corpus callosum forms from front to back except for the **rostrum that forms last**, so partial agenesis always includes the rostrum and splenium.

L. Cells proliferate in the walls of the neural tube and form a pseudostratified columnar layer with **ventricular and subventricular zones** (precursors of neurons and glia). Processes of these cells go from the lumen to the external basement membrane forming the **marginal zone** with an underlying intermediate zone. Most cells proliferate in the ventricular zone and migrate outward by ameboid movement guided by glial processes that extend from the ventricular zone to the **pial surface of**

the marginal zone. The migration is dictated by CAMs, ICAMs, and integrins (cell surface receptors). The cells mature, selectively die, group together, and form connections.

M. Brain stem—forms between 2 to 6 months. The **basal plate** has (medial to lateral) somatic efferent, special visceral efferent, and general visceral efferent nuclei. The **alar plate** has (medial to lateral in the plate and lateral to medial in the final position) general visceral afferent, special visceral afferent, and somatic afferent nuclei. Both efferent and afferent somatic nuclei are the most medial of their groups in the full-term human.

N. Spinal cord—has a **sulcus limitans** that forms between the dorsal (alar) and ventral (basal) plates. The connections form at 2 to 4 months.

O. Caudal spinal cord—forms separately by **retrograde differentiation** at 4 to 8 weeks as the caudal cell mass forms and cavitates.

P. **Neural crest**—the group of cells at the neural tube/somatic ectoderm junction. It forms portions of the **leptomeninges** (although the arachnoid part is of mesodermal origin), **Schwann cells**, craniospinal and sympathetic **ganglia** (and the **adrenal medulla**), **melanocytes** (i.e., the pigmented layer of the retina), and **APUD cells.**

Q. Ectodermal placodes (overlying the neural tube)—form the olfactory epithelium and the ganglia of cranial nerves V and VIII–X.

R. **Notocord** remnants—form the **nucleus pulposus** of the intervertebral discs. They are also believed to be the cells of origin of **chordomas.**

S. Dura and arachnoid—formed from **mesodermal** elements, and the pia is formed from **neuroectoderm.**

T. Full-term brain—weighs 400 g and is 90% water (the adult brain is 70% water). It has larger nuclei with less arborization. The anterior and lateral corticospinal tracts are incompletely myelinated. The corpus callosum and the fornix are completely unmyelinated. There may be myelination glia where immature oligodendrocytes in the site of myelination may appear like reactive astrocytes. There frequently is a cavum septum pellucidum. The immature cells around the lateral ventricles and the external granular layer of the cerebellum are gone after 12 to 15 months.

IV. DEVELOPMENTAL PATHOLOGY

A. Malformation—occurs when an organ is not formed properly. Dysplasia occurs when a tissue is not formed properly. Developmental injury may be caused by genetic abnormalities, chromosomal aberrations, or environmental factors (infections, drugs, chemicals, malnutrition, and maternal illness).

B. Neural tube defects (dysraphism)—caused by failure of fusion of the neural tube.

1. During neurulation (occurs at 17 to 30 days)—failure of fusion produces open defects by failure of disjunction of the neural and cutaneous ectoderm. The risk is increased with a neural tube defect in a sibling or a maternal folate deficiency. Maternal serum alfafetoprotein (AFP) is usually increased. This group includes spina bifida aperta, meningomyelocele, myelocele, anencephaly, and cranioschises.

2. Post neurulation (occurs at 26 to 60 days, or even near birth)—failure of fusion produces closed-skin–covered deficits such as spina bifida occulta, holoprosencephaly, encepaholoceles,

hydrocephalus, diastematomyelia, lipoma, meningocele, and Chiari malformations (**Fig. 2**).

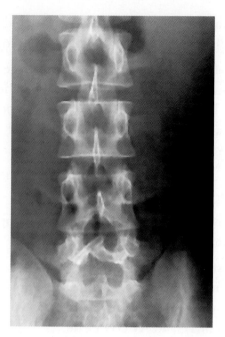

Figure 2   Spina bifida occulta; AP lumbar spine x-ray film demonstrates the L5 bifid spinous process.

3. Anencephaly—barely developed brain. It is the **most common congenital malformation**. It occurs in 0.03 to 0.7% of births in the United States and most commonly affects Caucasian females. Ninety-five percent of cases occur without a family history of neural tube defects. After one affected child, the risk increases to 2 to 5%. It is caused by chromosomal abnormalities or mechanical problems from adhesions to the placenta. The risk is increased with twins, polyhydramnios, hyperthermia, and **decreased maternal folate, zinc, or copper**. The neonates tend to be stillborn or to die within 2 months. They may have brain stem activity. Anencephaly is associated with the absence of scalp and skull. The brain consists of an exposed mass of tissue with an **area cerebrovascula** containing vessels, neural tissue, choroid, optic nerves, eyes, some cranial nerves, and brain stem. Craniorachischisis totalis occurs when the entire neuroaxis is involved. Fifteen to 40% have other organ malformations. Amniotic fluid has increased **AFP** and **acetylcholinesterase**.

4. Myelomeningocele—unfused spinal cord and meninges. It occurs in 0.07% of births in the United States and is more common in **females**. It is related to genetic and environmental factors. Risk factors include parental consanguinity, affected siblings, **decreased vitamin A or folate**, and use of valproic acid or carbamozipine (Tegretol). It is usually in the lumbar spine, with absent arachnoid and adjacent hydromyelia. It is associated with Chiari II malformations (100%), hydrocephalus (80%), lipoma (75%), syrinx (50%), diastematomyelia (40%), scoliosis (20%), kyphosis (10%), and orthopedic deformities and callosal dysgenesis (**Fig. 3**).

5. Meningocele—10% as common as myelomeningocele and has no gender predilection. It is **rarely associated with other anomalies** and is covered with skin. It consists of a pouching of dura through unfused bone.

6. Cephaloceles—include meningocele and meningoencephalocele. In the United States, they are occipital (80%), parietal (10%), frontal (10%), and rarely basal. They consist of an out-pouching of dura with or without neural tissue through unfused bone.

    (a) Occipital cephalocele—the **most frequent among Caucasians** and in Europe and North America. There is a female predilection. The cephalocele protrudes between the foramen magnum and the lambdoid suture. It is associated with myelomeningocele (7%), diastematomyelia (3%), Chiari II and III malformations, Dandy-Walker malformation, and Klippel-Feil syndrome (**Fig. 4**).

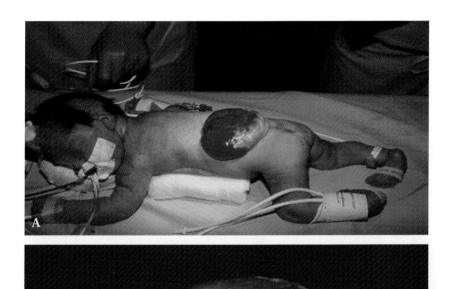

Figure 3 Myelomeningocoele. (A) Neural placode noted on center of dorsal aspect; (B) close-up image.

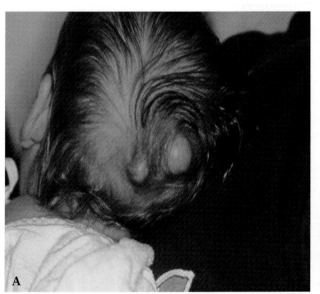

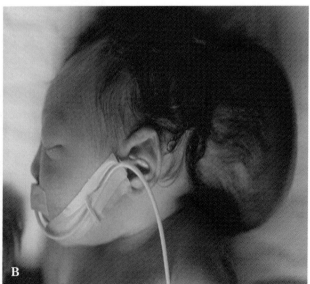

Figure 4 Encephaloceles. (A) Two small occipital encephaloceles; (B) large occipital encephalocele.

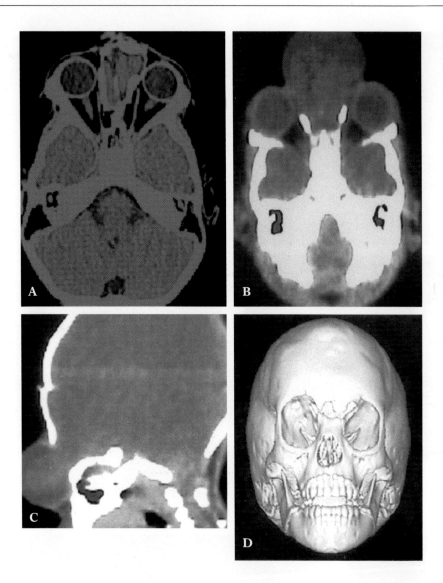

Figure 5 Nasofrontal encephalocele. Axial CTs and reconstructions (A to D) demonstrate a nasofrontal encephalocele.

(b) Parietal cephalocele—accounts for 10% of cases in the United States. There is a male predilection. The cephalocele protrudes between the lambda and bregma. It is associated with midline anomalies, agenesis of the corpus callosum, lobar holoprosencephaly, Dandy-Walker malformation, and Chiari II malformations.

(c) Transphenoidal cephalocele—rare, associated with sellar abnormalities, endocrine dysfunction, and agenesis of the corpus callosum.

(d) Sincipital (frontoethmoidal) cephalocele—the **most frequent type in Southeast Asia** and Australian aborigines. There is a male predilection. The cephalocele protrudes between the nasal and ethmoid bones and is not associated with neural tube defects.

(e) Sphenoethmoidal (nasal) cephalocele—the crista galli is absent or eroded and the foramen cecum is enlarged. The dural diverticulum normally regresses, but if it does not, it may form a dermal sinus tract. They are associated with dermoids and epidermoids and **nasal gliomas** (dysplastic or heterotopic glial tissue). If the crista galli is split, there is likely to be a dermoid present (**Fig. 5**).

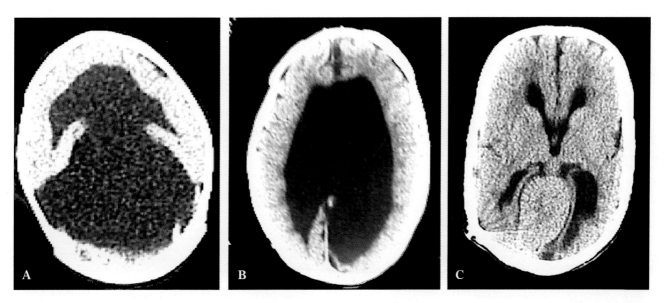

Figure 6   Holoprosencephaly. Axial CTs demonstrate alobar (A), semilobar (B), and lobar (C) holoprosencephaly with progressively more cleavage. The lobar variety has gray matter extending over the corpus callosum connecting the hemispheres.

       (f) Meckel's syndrome—cystic dysplastic kidneys, cardiac anomalies, orofacial clefting, and cephaloceles.

   7. Dermal sinus tracts—epithelium-lined tracts caused by faulty segmental disjunction. Sixty percent extend from the skin to the spinal canal, although they may end in the subcutaneous tissue, dura, spinal cord, or nerve roots. Fifty percent end in epidermoids or dermoids. More than 50% are lumbar and the next most frequent site is occipital. There is no gender predilection. Symptoms are mainly a result of **infection**. They are associated with skin dimples, hyperpigmentation, hairy nevi, and capillary malformations.

C. Cleavage disorders ("the face predicts the brain")—the cleavage of the telencephalon and the development of midline facial structures are dictated by the prechordal mesoderm.

   1. Holoprosencephaly (**Fig. 6**)

       (a) Alobar—completely undivided forebrain, **severe craniofacial abnormalities** (i.e., cyclopia), absence of olfactory nerves, abnormal optic nerves, monoventricle, fused basal ganglia and thalamus, absence of corpus callosum, septum pellucidum, falx, and fornix. It is associated with trisomy 13, 14, 15 and 18, polydactaly, renal dysplasia, and maternal diabetes.

       (b) Semilobar—monoventricle with forebrain divided by **partial falx and interhemispheric fissure**, partially separated thalamus and basal ganglia, and variable craniofacial abnormalities (i.e., hypotelorism and cleft lip).

       (c) Lobar—squared frontal horns, absence of the septum pellucidum, falx and interhemispheric fissure are present, and hemispheres are separated by thalamus and basal ganglia. There is **gray matter that extends across the midline** over the corpus callosum and there are **no craniofacial abnormalities**.

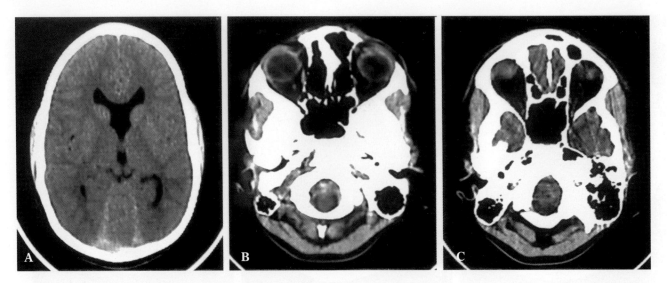

Figure 7   Septo-optic dysplasia. Axial CTs demonstrate absence of the septum pellucidum (A) and thin optic nerves (B and C).

2. Arrhinencephaly—the absence of the olfactory bulbs and tracts with normal cortex and gray matter in place of the corpus callosum. It is associated with holoprosencephaly and **Kallman's syndrome** (anosmia, hypogonadism, and mental retardation).

3. Septo-optic dysplasia (de Morsier's syndrome)—occurs with mild lobar holoprosencephaly, absence of the septum pellucidum, schizencephaly, and hypoplastic optic nerves. It is associated with seizures, visual symptoms, hypothalamic-pituitary dysfunction (precocious puberty), enlarged ventricles, and hypotelorism (**Fig. 7**).

4. Cleidocranial dysostosis—occurs with retention of mandibular teeth, delayed closure of fontanelles, wormian bones, and midline defects.

D. Migrational disorders

1. Heterotopias—normal neurons in abnormal CNS locations (i.e., in the centrum semiovale, along the lateral ventricles, or in the cerebellar white matter). They may be laminar or nodular and usually do not enhance (**Fig. 8**).

2. Ectopias—neurons in locations brain tissue should not be in (i.e., the subarachnoid space). They are associated with dysraphism and hydranencephaly.

3. Lissencephaly—smooth brain. In the complete form, the cerebral hemispheres have no sulci. In the incomplete form, there are several shallow sulci. It is associated with in-utero infections.

4. Pachygyria—overall decreased number of gyri and those that are present are enlarged.

5. Polymicrogyria—wrinkled-appearing brain with many small gyri. It forms occasionally after neuronal migration from neural injury. Usually there are only four layers of cortex in the abnormal gyri. It may be focal or widespread.

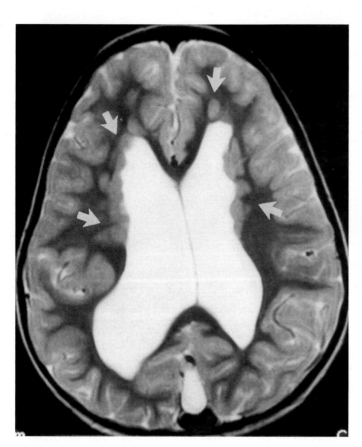

Figure 8   Gray matter heterotopia.

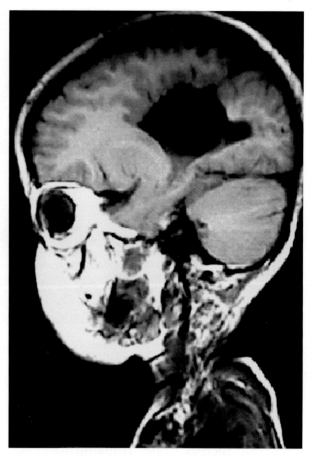

Figure 9   Schizencephaly. Sagittal T1-weighted MRI demonstrates gray matter–lined cleft extending from the subarachnoid space to the lateral ventricle.

6. Schizencephaly—a **gray matter–lined** cleft extending from the pia to the ventricle. The cleft may be filled with CSF (opened lip) or collapsed (closed lip) (**Fig. 9**).

7. Porencephaly—a cleft **not lined with gray matter**, but by gliotic white matter that forms after an insult to an otherwise normal brain.

8. Unilateral megaencephaly—hamartomatous overgrowth of one hemisphere with ipsilaterally enlarged ventricle and cortex. It is associated with neuronal migration disorders.

9. Agenesis of the corpus callosum—the corpus callosum forms from anterior to posterior, but the rostrum forms last so the **splenium and rostrum are almost always involved with agenesis**. Agenesis may be complete or partial. It is characterized by a high-riding third ventricle, radial spokelike gyri, **Probst's bundles** (longitudinal white matter tracts indenting the medial ventricles), and colpocephaly. Occasionally, the cingulate gyrus, anterior commissure, or fornix may be absent. **Fifty percent have associated abnormalities**

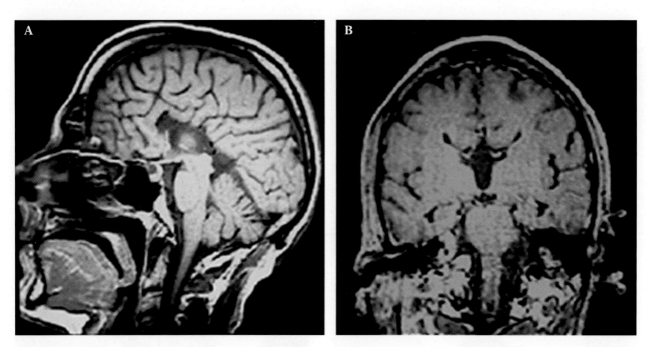

Figure 10   Agenesis of the corpus callosum. T1-weighted sagittal (A) and coronal (B) MRIs demonstrating absence of the corpus callosum with characteristic "Viking helmet" ventricles.

such as Chiari II malformations, Dandy-Walker malformations, migrational disorders, cephaloceles, holoprosencephaly, lipomas, and azygous anterior cerebral arteries. **Aicardi's syndrome** has a female predominance and consists of callosal agenesis, ocular abnormalities, and infantile spasms (**Fig. 10**).

E. Other developmental syndromes

1. Congenital hydrocephalus—commonly due to aqueductal stenosis, chiari II malformation, Dandy-Walker malformation, infection, and intraventricular hemorrhage.

2. Chiari I malformation (**Fig. 11**)—peglike tonsils extending below the foramen magnum (6 mm under the foramen magnum at age < 10 years, 5 mm < 30 years, 4 mm < 80 years, and 3 mm < 90 years). If the tonsils extend > 12 mm below the foramen magnum, all are symptomatic, and from 5 to 10 mm, 70% are symptomatic. Chiari I malformation occasionally forms after frequent lumbar punctures or placement of a lumboperitoneal shunt. Chiari I malformation is **not associated with other brain abnormalities** but is associated with **skeletal abnormalities** in 25% of cases: basilar invagination (25 to 50%), Klippel-Feil syndrome with fused cervical vertebrae (5 to 10%), atlanto-occipital fusion (5%), and cervical spina bifida occulta (5%). It presents in early **adulthood** and symptoms include **pain**, occipital headache, Lhermitte's sign, long tract signs, **syringomyelia** (20 to 40%, although 60 to 90% of symptomatic cases), and hydrocephalus (25%). Chiari malformations of all types present differently at different age groups.

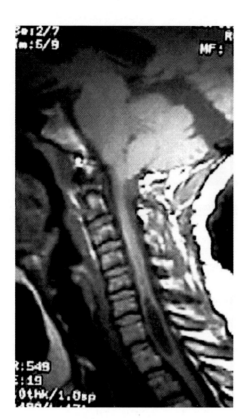

Figure 11   Chiari 1 malformation. Sagittal T1-weighted MRI demonstrates peglike tonsils extending below foramen magnum with an associated syrinx.

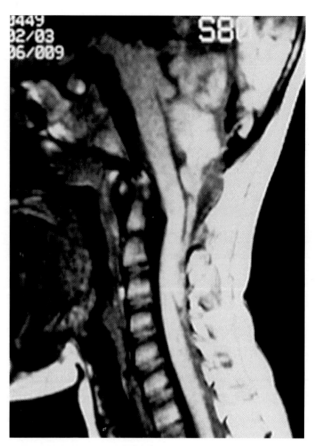

Figure 12   Chiari 2 (Arnold-Chiari) malformation. Sagittal T1-weighted MRI with tectal beaking, low-lying torcula, and vermian descent.

(a) Infants—hydrocephalus and brain stem compression with apnea, decreased gag reflex, nystagmus, and spasticity.

(b) Children—nystagmus, spastic paralysis, and bulbar dysfunction.

(c) Adolescents—progressive spasticity and capelike pain and temperature loss in the upper limbs.

(d) Adults—occipital headache, neck and arm pain, and nystagmus (**Fig. 11**).

3. Chiari II malformation (Arnold-Chiari malformation)—thought to develop when the neural folds do not completely meet and there is abnormal ventricular CSF flow into the amnion with collapse of the ventricles. A small posterior fossa develops and as the cerebellum grows, it herniates upward forming a large tentorial incisura and it herniates downward pushing the vermis and brain stem through the foramen magnum. It presents in neonates and is associated with many abnormalities (**Fig. 12**).

(a) Skull and dura—lacunar skull ("**lukenschadel**," with scooped out appearance), small posterior fossa, **low-lying torcula** and transverse sinus, large foramen magnum,

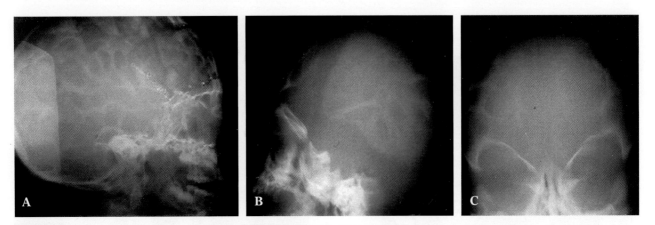

Figure 13   Lukenschadel skull. Lateral (A and B) and AP (C) skull x-ray films demonstrate the "copper beading" or scooped-out appearance with myelomeningocoele.

concave petrous temporal bones, short concave clivus, and a thin falx cerebri with occasional interdigitating gyri through fenestrations in the falx cerebri (**Fig. 13**).

(b) Hindbrain—**herniation of the vermis**, nodulus, uvula, and pyramis through the foramen magnum, **medullary kinking** (70%), enhancing ectopic choroid, upward cerebellar herniation, and **tectal beaking**.

(c) CSF spaces—tubular fourth ventricle, large third ventricle with **enlarged massa intermedia**, colpocephaly (large atria and occipital horns), aqueductal stenosis, small cisterna magna, and **hydrocephalus** (90%).

(d) Cerebral hemispheres—heterotopias, polymicrogyria, and callosal dysgenesis.

(e) Spine—**myelomeningocele** (100%), syrinx (50 to 90%), diastematomyelia, and incomplete C1 arch (70%). It is not associated with lipomyelomeningocele.

4. Chiari III malformation—hindbrain herniation into an encephalocele, usually occipital or high cervical (**Fig. 14**).

5. Chiari IV malformation—cerebellar hypoplasia.

6. Dandy-Walker malformation—**posterior fossa cyst continuous** with the fourth ventricle with partial or complete **vermian absence**. It may be due to failure of development of the superior medullary velum (roof of the fourth ventricle) combined with fourth ventricle outlet atresia. It is associated with a large posterior fossa, **high tentorium** and transverse sinus, lambdoid-torcula inversion, hydrocephalus (80%), callosal agenesis (25%), heterotopias, schizencephaly, cephaloceles, dolicocephaly, **cardiac abnormalities**, and **polydactyly** (**Fig. 15**).

7. Dandy-Walker variant—mild inferior vermian hypoplasia with open communication between the fourth ventricle and the cisterna magna through an enlarged vallecula. The fourth ventricle is enlarged but the posterior fossa is normal size. There is no associated hydrocephalus.

8. Mega cisterna magna—posterior fossa CSF accumulation in an enlarged cisterna magna. There is a normal fourth ventricle and no hydrocephalus. It fills with intrathecal contrast.

9. Posterior fossa arachnoid cyst—posterior fossa CSF accumulation with a normal cerebellum and fourth ventricle. There may or may not be hydrocephalus. The cyst does not fill with intrathecal contrast.

10. Lhermitte-Duclos disease—hypertrophied cerebellar granular cell layer neurons and increased myelin in the molecular layer of the cerebellum with thick folia. There is mass effect on the fourth ventricle. There may be calcifications, hydrocephalus, and folia with increased signal intensity on

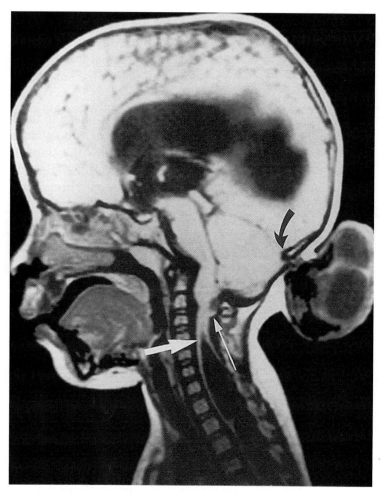

Figure 14   Chiari 3 malformation (occipital encephalocoele).

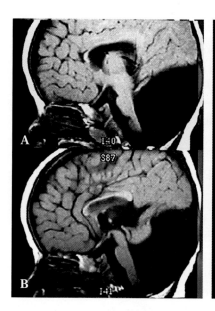

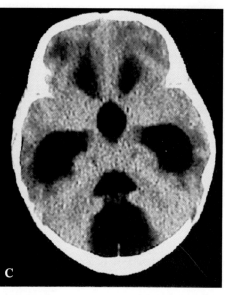

Figure 15   Dandy-Walker malformation. Sagittal T1-weighted MRIs (A and B) and axial CT (C) demonstrate vermian agenesis and connection of fourth ventricle to posterior fossa cyst.

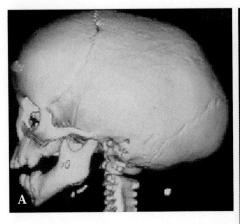

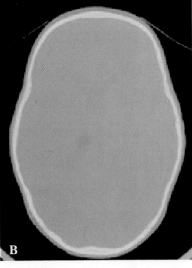

Figure 16   Sagittal synostosis (scapho-cephaly, dolicocephaly). CT reconstruction (A) and axial CT (B).

T2-weighted MRI. It is associated with megaencephaly, polydactyly, giantism, heterotopias, and cutaneous hemangiomas.

11. Hydromyelia—a distended central canal of the spinal cord **lined by ependymal cells**. It is associated with Chiari II malformations and myelomeningoceles.

12. Syringomyelia—a fluid-filled cavity in the spinal cord lined by astrocytes.

13. Syringobulbia—a fluid-filled cavity extending into the brain stem.

14. Fetal alcohol syndrome—characterized by growth retardation, craniofacial dysmorphism, CNS and visceral malformations, mental retardation, and **microcephaly**. It is associated with migrational defects, hydrocephalus, schizencephaly, callosal agenesis, and neural tube defects. The incidence is increased if mothers use drugs, have poor nutrition, or smoke tobacco.

15. Colpocephaly—dilated occipital horns associated with agenesis of the corpus callosum and periventricular leukomalacia, mental retardation, and seizures.

16. Craniosynostosis—premature fusion of the sutures causing abnormal skull growth and shape. Surgical treatment to open the sutures and reshape as needed is best done between 3–6 months and is generally performed for cosmetic purposes.

    (a) Sagittal synostosis—**most common** (50%), male predominance, causes scaphocephaly or dolicocephaly (**Fig. 16**).

    (b) Unilateral coronal synostosis—25%, causes anterior plagiocephaly, female predominance (**Fig. 17**).

    (c) Bilateral coronal synostosis—usually genetic, causes brachicephaly, associated with Apert's and Crouzon's syndromes (**Fig. 18**).

    (d) Unilateral lambdoidal synostosis—1.3%, male predominance, causes posterior plagiocephaly, also may be due to the baby lying on one side too often. This is treated initially by changing the infant's sleeping position, not by surgery (**Fig. 19**).

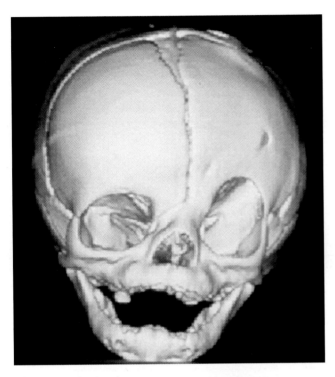

Figure 17   Unilateral coronal synostosis (plagiocephaly). CT reconstruction with "harlequin eye" on the left.

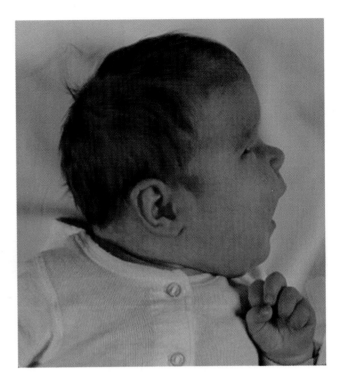

Figure 18   Brachycephaly; bilateral coronal synostosis.

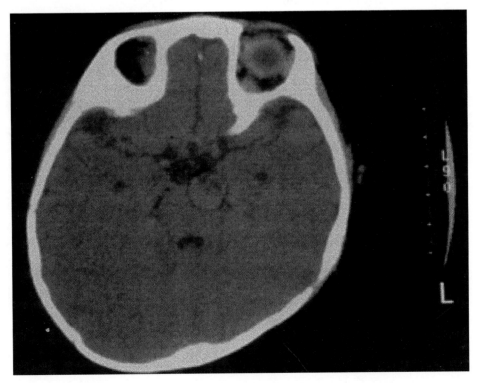

Figure 19   Lambdoidal synostosis (plagiocephaly); axial CT.

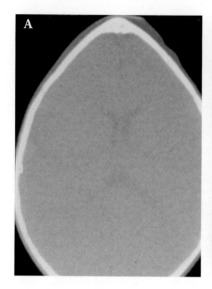 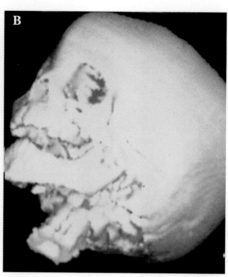

Figure 20   Metopic synostosis (trigono-cephaly); axial CT (A) and CT reconstruction (B).

(e) Metopic synostosis—5%, causes **trigonocephaly (Fig. 20)**.

(f) Turricephaly—5 to 10%, synostosis of both coronal sutures and the sphenofrontal sutures, causes a tall broad head.

(g) Oxycephaly—5 to 10%, synostosis of multiple sutures, causes a cone-shaped head.

(h) Pansynostosis—causes Lukenschadel head.

(i) **Crouzon's syndrome—most frequent** craniofacial syndrome, **autosomal dominant** or sporadic inheritance, shallow orbits, exophthalamos, midface hypoplasia, malformed ears, agenesis of the corpus callosum, less severe mental retardation than with Apert's syndrome, and **increased incidence of hydrocephalus**. More than one suture is involved, and they may have oxycephaly, turricephaly, or dolicocephaly. The sphenofrontal synostosis produces exophthalmus.

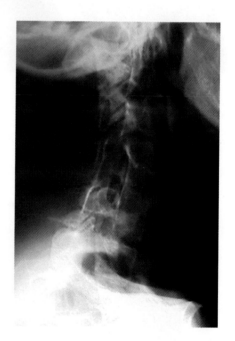

Figure 21   Klippel-Feil syndrome.

(j) **Apert's syndrome**—second most common craniofacial syndrome, **autosomal dominant** or sporadic inheritance, turricephalic head, maxillary hypoplasia, orbital hypertelorism, **syndactyly**, **mental retardation**, deafness, flat nose, and vertebral and skeletal abnormalities. Only the coronal suture is involved. There are **GI, GU, and cardiac abnormalities** and increased incidence of frontal encephaloceles.

17. Klippel-Feil syndrome—congenital **fusion of the upper cervical vertebrae**, associated with **Sprengel's deformity** (elevation of the scapula) and Chiari I malformation (**Fig. 21**).

F. Chromosomal disorders

1. Trisomy 13 (Pateau's syndrome)—female predominance, **hypotelorism**, holoprosencephaly, microcephaly, microphthalmia, **cleft palate and lip**, **polydactyly**, **dextrocardia**, and ocular abnormalities. Death ensues before 9 months.

2. Trisomy 18 (Edward's syndrome)—female predominance, gyral dysplasia, callosal agenesis, Chiari II malformation, dolicocephaly, cerebellar hypoplasia, **hypertelorism**, microphthalmos, syndactyly, and ventricular septal defects. Less than 10% live 1 year.

3. Trisomy 21 (Down syndrome)—most frequent of the chromosomal abnormalities and occurs in 0.1% of births. Varieties include (1) sporadic trisomy (95%) (increased risk with maternal age > 35 years), (2) Robertson translocation 21q and 14 or 21q and 22q in 4% (not associated with age), and (3) mosaic (1%). It is characterized by brachycephaly, **hypotelorism**, hypoplastic maxilla and nose, skull base abnormalities, cervical stenosis, atlantoaxial instability, underdeveloped inferior temporal gyrus, narrow superior temporal gyrus, flattened occipital pole, mental retardation, lens opacities, **congenital heart disease** (increased risk of brain abscess), and **Alzheimer's disease** (by 40 years).

4. 5p deletion (cri du chat syndrome)—mental retardation, microcephaly, **hypertelorism**, and congenital heart disease.

5. 15q deletion (Prader-Willi syndrome)—mental retardation, truncal obesity, short stature, and hypogonadism.

6. Fragile X syndrome—**the most frequent hereditary mental retardation**. It has a male predominance, although one-third are female (these have a normal IQ). There is a dysmorphic appearance with long face, large testicles, and vermian hypoplasia.

7. Ataxia-telangiectasia—cerebellar atrophy, lentiform nucleus calcifications, pachygyria, impaired immune system, increased lymphoreticular carcinoma, and defective DNA repair.

V. PERINATAL BRAIN INJURIES

A. Perinatal brain injury—may be caused by birth or other trauma, infection, metabolic disorders, or maternal intoxications.

B. Caput succedaneum—cutaneous hemorrhagic edema in the skin over the calvarium caused by pressure during birth with vascular stasis. It crosses sutures and resolves in 48 hours.

C. Subaponeurotic hemorrhage—blood accumulates under the aponeurosis.

D. Cephalohematoma—subperiosteal blood that **does not cross suture lines**. It is usually parietal and may calcify.

E. Epidural hematoma (EDH)—rare, associated with fractures.

F. Intradural hematoma—either falcine or tentorial and associated with asphyxia or mechanical trauma. It rarely has clinical significance.

G. Subdural hematoma (SDH)—rare, caused by mechanical trauma from a small birth canal, rapid or prolonged labor, abnormal presentation, premature birth with increased skull compliance, large head, and forceps deliveries. It forms from tearing of the bridging veins over the convexity, tentorium, or skull base (see Fig. 246C). Occipital osteodiastasis is the traumatic separation of the squamous and lateral occipital bone with tearing of the occipital sinus and bleeding in the posterior fossa. Laceration of the falx or inferior sagittal sinus causes bleeding over the corpus callosum.

H. Subarchnoid hemorrhage (SAH)—caused by hypoxia or trauma and usually has a good outcome.

I. Intraparenchymal hemorrhage—caused by coagulation defects, vitamin K deficiency, trauma, vascular malformation, tumor, or stroke.

J. Periventricular/intraventricular hemorrhage—occurs in 40% of births < 35 weeks and 3 to 7% of full-term births. There is increased incidence with **prematurity and acute respiratory distress syndrome (ARDS)**. It develops an average of **72 hours postpartum** in the subependymal **germinal matrix** near the foramen of Monro or the body of the caudate. **In full-term births, the hemorrhage develops in the choroid plexus of the lateral ventricle.** Mortality is 20 to 60% and morbidity is 15 to 40% (mainly motor deficits and mental retardation). Hydrocephalus may be by obstruction at the aqueduct, fourth ventricular outlet, or arachnoid granulations.

K. Delivery trauma—usually causes SDH (interhemispheric or tentorial) and less frequently posterior fossa SAH that results from the sudden fronto-occipital shortening that may tear a suture, sinus, or vein. The risk increases with cephalopelvic disproportion or abnormal presentation.

L. Hypoxic/ischemic perinatal brain injury

   1. Acute injury

      (a) Periventricular leukomalacia—increased incidence with prematurity, congenital heart disease, shock, sepsis, and respiratory distress syndrome. It occurs within 72 hours and causes lower extremity weakness and visual problems.

      (b) Gray matter necrosis—seen in full-term births with perinatal asphyxia and mainly affects the subthalamus, lateralgeniculate body (LGB), inferior colliculus, cranial nerves, dentate nuclei, Purkinje's cells, and the cortical internal granular layer.

   2. Chronic injury

      (a) Ulegyria—parieto-occipital mushroom-like atrophic gyri with atrophy in sulcus valleys.

      (b) Status marmoratus—the thalamus, neostriatum, and cortex develop irregular intersecting bands of myelin and astrocytic fibers that grossly resembles marble caused by cell loss followed by remyelination.

3. Kernicterus—caused by increased unbound **unconjugated bilirubin** staining the gray matter and causing neuronal necrosis. It affects predominantly the **GP**, thalamus, subthalamus, and CN III and VIII nuclei, causing symmetric cell loss with extrapyramidal motor signs. Treat the elevated bilirubin with phototherapy using ultraviolet light, but if the bilirubin is >20 or >15 with associated sepsis, prematurity, acidosis, or low albumin, treat with an exchange transfusion.

4. Cavitary encephalopathies—caused by infections, genetic defects, or toxic gases.

   (a) Porencephaly—a cavity that extends from the leptomeninges to the ventricles or superficial white matter lined by white matter (as opposed to schizencephaly, which is a cleft lined by gray matter).

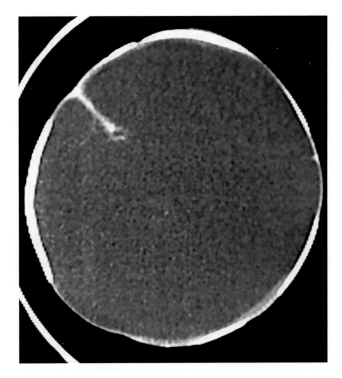

Figure 22   Hydranencephaly; axial CT demonstrates a very thin rim of brain.

   (b) Hydranencephaly—most or all of the cortex is replaced by CSF, may result from cerebral ischemia (internal carotid artery [ICA] occlusions) or infection (i.e., CMV or *Toxoplasma*) (**Fig. 22**).

   (c) Multicystic encephalopathy—anterior and middle cerebral artery distribution multiple cavities.

VI. INFECTIOUS DISEASES

A. Meningitis

   1. Etiologies—the most frequent pathogen overall is **H. influenza**, and the most frequent cause in adults is **S. pneumonia**. The subarachnoid space near the blood vessels fill first with neutrophils and fibrin, then macrophages, and then it eventually fibroses. Meningitis is associated with arteritis, phlebitis, superior sagittal sinus thrombosis, and hydrocephalus. The three most common causes of meningitis (*H. influenza*, *S. pneumonia*, and *N. meningitiditis*) all normally colonize the nasopharynx. The fourth most common pathogen is *Listeria*, which causes opportunistic infections. *S. aureus* is associated with postoperative infections and *S. epidermidis* is the most common cause of shunt infections. The mortality form various types of meningitis are 10% (*H. influenza* and *N. meningitiditis*), 25% (*S. pneumonia*), and 50% (neonatal, with 50% of survivors having permanent sequelae).

   2. Neonate (0 to 4 weeks)—the most frequent organisms are (1) **group B streptococcus** with acute onset <5 days postpartum with sepsis and pneumonia. It is associated with intrapartum

infection and has a 15 to 30% mortality; (2) *E. coli* is the most frequent cause in Latin America, especially with the K1 capsular antigen; and (3) *Listeria*. Sequelae include hydrocephalus, encephalomalacia at the border zones and in the white matter, seizures, deafness, mental retardation, and focal deficits. The overall morbidity and mortality is 30 to 50%. Risk increases with prematurity, prolonged membrane rupture, traumatic delivery, congenital malformations (myelomeningoceole or dermal sinus), and acquired respiratory, gastro-intestinal (GI), and umbilical infections.

3. Four to 12 weeks—the most common pathogen is **S. pneumonia**.

4. Three months to 3 years: The most common pathogen is **H. influenza**, although it rarely occurs after 5 years; 85% are type b. It develops from nasopharyngeal colonization that leads to sepsis followed by meningitis. Blood cultures are positive in 70%. The bacteria needs X and V growth factors to grow. It is associated with **bilateral subdural effusions** (usually culture negative because they are due to increased permeability of blood vessels and also related to *S. Pneumonia* infections) and frequently causes seizures. Treatment is with third-generation cephalosporins. Concomitant use of **steroids** has been shown to decrease the incidence of deafness in children.

5. Children and young adults—the most frequent pathogen is **N. meningitiditis**, and the meningitis occurs in epidemics. It develops from nasopharygeal colonization that leads to hematologic dissemination and meningitis. The risk increases with decreased complement and in patients with systemic lupus erythromatosis (SLE). It is associated with cutaneous eruptions (60%), arteritis, and cardiac deaths. The Waterhouse-Friderichsen syndrome is meningococcemia with vasomotor collapse, shock, disseminated intravascular coagulation (DIC), and diffuse hemorrhages, especially in the adrenal glands. *N. meningitiditis* is a gram-negative intracellular diplococcus. Treatment is with penicillin or chloramphenicol.

6. Elderly—the most common pathogen is **S. pneumonia**. It is more common in the elderly (because of age-dependent immune decline) and alcoholics (ethanol induces a chemotaxis defect and impairs phagocytosis). Risk is increased with trauma (it is the normal flora of the mastoid, ear, sinus, and nose), infection, and sickle cell disease (caused by impaired splenic filtering, the risk is not increased in adults). Detection uses the Quellung reaction. Treatment is with penicillin.

B. Brain abscess (**Fig. 23**)

1. Etiologies—the most common pathogen is **Streptococcus** and the most common cause is adjacent ear or sinus infection (40%), with spreading along the valveless venous channels (frontal sinus to frontal lobe, sphenoid sinus to temporal lobe, and ear to cerebellum or temporal lobe). Thirty-three percent are from hematogenous spread from another infected site (usually lung, dental disease, or trauma more likely multiple; and usually in the **distal middle cerebral artery (MCA) territory at the gray/white junction**); 20% have an unknown cause.

2. Risk—increases with cyanotic heart disease (5% incidence of brain abscesses, accounts for 60% of abscesses in children, and is due to decreased pulmonary blood filtration and lower oxygen tension in the brain) and **pulmonary arterio-venus malformations (AVMs)** (5% incidence of abscesses, associated with Rendu Osler Weber syndrome).

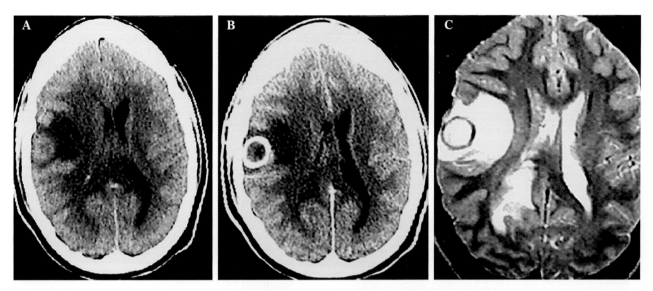

Figure 23   Brain abscess. Noninfused (A) and infused (B) CTs demonstrate a smooth ring-enhancing lesion, and T2-weighted MRI (C) demonstrates the associated edema.

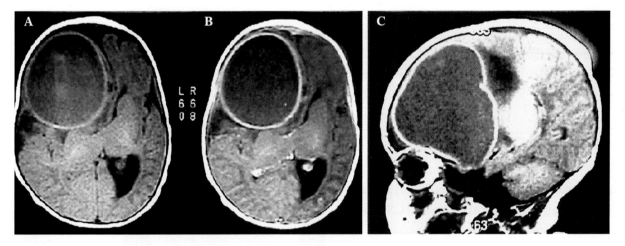

Figure 24   Neonatal brain abscess. Axial T1-weighted noninfused (A) and infused (B) MRIs and infused sagittal T1-weighted MRI (C) demonstrates a massive cystic abscess cavity.

3.   Neonates—the most common causes are ***Citrobacter***, ***Bacteroides***, ***Proteus***, and gram-negative bacilli (**Fig. 24**).

4.   Trauma—the most frequent cause is Staphylococcus, and with otitis, enteric bacilli are common.

5.   Subacute bacterial endocarditis (SBE)—with streptococcal deposits on the valves usually causes ischemic strokes, but not abscesses. 10% of SBE cases have a mycotic aneurysm develop. Acute endocarditis caused by Staphylococcus or hemolytic Streptococcus may cause multiple abscesses. There are mixed species in 30%.

6.   Brain abscesses occur most commonly at the gray-white junction and are multiple in 35%. The abscess has a tendency to **rupture into the ventricle** because the capsule is thinner medially where there is decreased collagen formation. This has been postulated to be due to increased oxygen content near the cortex that stimulates the fibroblasts to develop. The mortality is 5% and is mainly from brain herniation or abscess rupture into the ventricles.

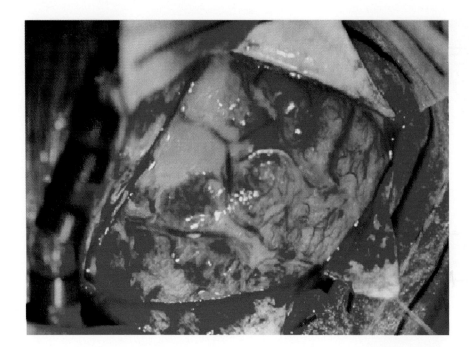

Figure 25   Subdural empyema; thick pus collection over the convexity.

7. Pathologic stages—(a) early cerebritis (up to 5 days), (b) late cerebritis (5 days to 2 weeks); (c) early capsule formation (2 to 3 weeks); and (d) late capsule formation (>3 weeks, there is a firm capsule around the abscess).

C. Encephalitis—commonly by *Legionella* (CSF culture is usually negative), *Mycoplasma*, *Listeria* (in neonates and immunosuppresed, CSF culture is usually positive), and *Brucella*.

D. Subdural empyema—mainly caused by **Streptococcus** and *Bacteroides* from an adjacent infection. Treat with antibiotics and drainage with multiple burr holes or an osteoplastic flap. Consider antibiotic therapy alone if asymptomatic (**Fig. 25**).

E. Epidural abscess—most commonly caused by **S. aureus**, *Streptococcus*, gram-negative bacilli, and tuberculosis. It is usually secondary to an associated osteomyelitis or sinusitis and most frequently occurs in the thoracic, lumbar, or sacral spine (**Fig. 26**).

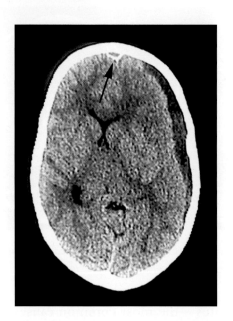

Figure 26   Epidural abscess and subdural empyema. Infused CT demonstrates a large convexity low-density subdural collection and a small anterior rim-enhancing epidural lesion (arrow).

F. Osteomyelitis—most commonly caused by the same lesions as epidural abscesses and occurs with sinusitis (**Fig. 27**), after craniotomy, or by hematologic spread. It is characterized by moth-eaten cortical bone with poor margins and soft tissue swelling. X-ray films may appear similar to metastatic lesions. **Gradenigo's syndrome** is petrous apex osteomyelitis with CN VI palsy and retro-orbital pain and may occur in children from extension of severe otitis.

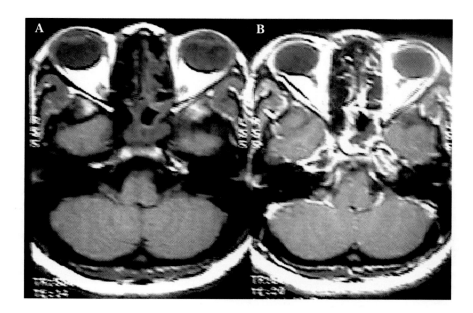

Figure 27   Sphenoid sinusitis. Axial non-infused (A) and infused (B) T1-weighted MRIs demonstrating thickened enhancing mucosa.

VII. INFECTIOUS PATHOGENS

A. Mycobacterial infections

    1. Tuberculosis (TB)—caused by *Mycobacterium tuberculosis*.

        (a) Cerebrospinal fluid (CSF) evaluation—increased lymphocytes, decreased glucose (but not as low as with pyogenic infections), and increased protein up to 200 mg/dL. Acid-fast bacilli are seen in the CSF in <25% of cases and require up to 4 weeks to grow in culture. It is diagnosed by positive PPD and TB lesions found elsewhere in the body. Two-thirds of cases have active TB infections elsewhere in the body. Treatment is with 24 months of triple antibiotics.

        (b) TB meningitis—characterized by a thick **basilar** exudate, small miliary granulomas on the convexities, and frequent vascular occlusions. The morbidity is 80% and the mortality is 30%. It usually results from hematogenous spread. Pathologic examination **(Fig. 28)** demonstrates granulomas with **caseating necrosis**, lymphocytes, and **Langhan's giant cells**.

        (c) Tuberculomas—in the brain parenchyma are rare in the United States but are common intracranial masses in other countries such as India and Mexico. They may be solid or cystic, 30% are multiple, and in children two-thirds are infratentorial.

        (d) Miliary TB—has innumerable small lesions, is rare, and is more frequently seen in children.

    2. Leprosy—caused by *Mycobacterium leprae*. It most frequently occurs in tropical climates, California, Texas, New York, and Louisiana. In the United States it is primarily brought in by travelers. There are two types:

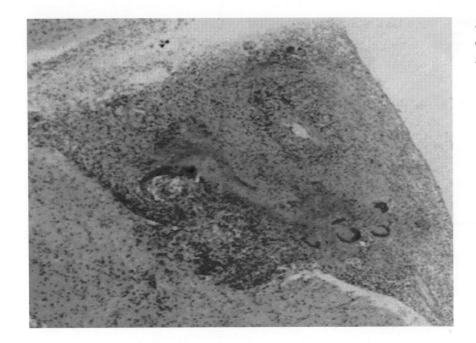

Figure 28   Tuberculous meningitis (H and E); caseating granuloma with Langhans' giant cells.

    (a) Lepromatous form—seen with low host resistance and has lepra cells that are plump histiocytes filled with organisms. Lesions are located in the skin on cooler parts of the body (i.e., hands, feet, head, peripheral nerves, anterior eyes, upper airways, and testes). The lepromin skin test is negative.

    (b) Tuberculoid form—seen with maximal host resistance and there are areas of hypesthetic skin, inflamed swollen nerves, caseating granulomas, and occasional gram-negative bacilli seen on histologic examination. The lepromin skin test is positive.

B. Other granulomatous disease

    1. Sarcoid—systemic granulomatous disease of unknown cause that involves lymph nodes (especially hilar), lungs, skin, eyes, salivary glands, and liver. The nervous system is involved in **5%** of cases with cranial nerve palsies (**especially CN VII**), aseptic meningitis, pituitary dysfunction, hydrocephalus, and noncaseating granulomas at the **base of the brain** (especially, the **hypothalamus**). It may also cause myelopathy, neuropathy, and myopathy. Sarcoid is most common in African-Americans. The serum angiotensin-converting enzyme (ACE) level is usually elevated. Treatment is with steroids (See Fig. 155).

    2. Whipple's disease—a chronic multisystem disease caused by *Tropheryma whippelii*. It is characterized by weight loss, abdominal pain, diarrhea, lymphadenopathy, arthralgia, and Alzheimer's disease–like neurologic symptoms (10%). Pathologic examination demonstrates foamy macrophages with **PAS-positive granules**. These are degenerating bacilli. Treat with tetracycline.

C. Spirochetes

    1. Neurosyphilis—a sexually transmitted disease caused by *Treponema pallidum*. A genital lesion (chancre) forms 3 weeks after infection, and secondary lesions develop several weeks later. Twenty-five percent of cases involve the CNS, but usually after 3 years. Treatment is with penicillin and CSF testing at 6 months and 1 year for evaluation of treatment success. There are four types of neurosyphilis:

(a) Meningovascular syphilis (lues)—occurs after 7 years and is characterized by subacute or chronic meningitis with perivascular lymphocytes, **Huebner's arteritis** with intimal proliferation and vessel obliteration, and multiple ischemic strokes in the basal ganglia and MCA territory.

(b) General paresis of the insane—occurs after 15 years and is characterized by invasion into the parenchyma with chronic encephalitis, atrophy, and gummas with nonsuppurative necrotic debris, progressive physical and mental deterioration, and Argyll Robertson pupils.

(c) **Tabes dorsalis**—occurs after 15 to 20 years and is characterized by myelopathy from meningeal fibrosis. There is mainly dorsal root and posterior column involvement, W-shaped demyelination in the **thoracic and lumbar** spinal cord from the posterior horns inward, lightning-like pains, sensory ataxia, urinary incontinence, decreased lower limb deep tendon reflexes (DTRs), decreased proprioception and vibratory sense, positive Rhomberg's test, **Argyll Robertson pupils** (90%), ptosis, optic atrophy, and **Charcot joints** of the hip, knee, and ankle.

(d) Congenital syphilis—includes **Hutchinson's triad** of notched teeth, deafness, and interstitial keratitis. This is also associated with meningovascular syphilis.

2. Lyme disease—caused by *Borrelia burgdorferi*, a **tickborne** spirochete and causes **erythema migrans** (70%). Fifteen percent have neurologic symptoms such as **aseptic meningitis**, cranial neuritis (especially CN VII), encephalitis, myelopathy, radiculopathy, and peripheral neuropathy. It is most frequently seen from May through July in New England, along the Pacific coast, and in Wisconsin and Minnesota. The symptoms are caused by immune complexes and vasculitis with a postviral-type demyelination and perivascular infiltration. Diagnosis is by ELISA and treatment is with tetracycline.

D. Other bacterial infections

1. Actinomyces—a branched filamentous bacteria that looks like a fungus. It is rare in the CNS, contains sulfur granules, and is AFB negative.

2. Nocardia—an opportunist that usually infects the lungs, although the CNS evaluation is involved in 30% of cases. It forms multiple abscesses and is AFB positive.

E. Fungal infections

1. Mycotic infections—usually occur in immunosuppressed patients and result from hematologic spread from the lungs. They cause **basilar meningitis** (with cranial neuropathies, hydrocephalus, and arteritis causing strokes) or abscesses with granulomas. CSF evaluation reveals increased lymphocytes and decreased glucose. All fungi stain with methenamine silver. The true pathogens are *Histoplasma*, *Blastomyces*, and *Coccidiomyces*; all of the others only infect the immunosuppressed.

2. Candidiasis—caused by *C. albicans*. It is the **most frequent CNS fungal infection**. *C. albicans* is normal flora of the GI tract, skin, and genitals. Risk of infection increases with antibiotics, steroids, IV lines, diabetes mellitus, burns, **immunosuppression**, and intravenous drug

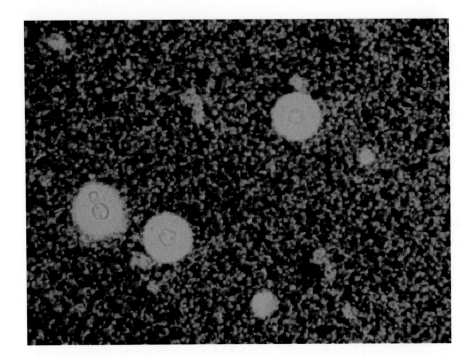

Figure 29   Cryptococcus (India ink); yeast organisms surrounded by clear halos.

abuse (IVDA). It forms multiple microabscesses with granulomas and rarely causes meningitis. It also infects the urine, blood, skin, heart, and lungs. Treatment is with amphotericin B.

3. Histoplasmosis—caused by *H. capsulatum* from the soil of the Ohio, Mississippi, and St. Lawrence river valleys. It frequently causes pulmonary infections and only rarely CNS infections with basilar meningitis and occasional parenchymal granulomas.

4. Blastomycosis—caused by *B. dermatidis* from the soil of the eastern United States. The CNS is involved in less than 5% of cases. Abscess is more frequent then meningitis. Culture demonstrates a single budding yeast.

5. Cryptococcosis—caused by *C. neoformans* from soil contaminated with **bird feces**. It is the **most frequent fungal meningitis** and the second most frequent CNS fungal infection. There are rarely cryptococcomas in the parenchyma. CSF cultures are positive (75%), cryptococcus antigen is positive (90%), and **India ink stain is positive (Fig. 29)** (50%), with a single budding yeast with a thick capsule. The capsule disappears during the tissue preparation to form the characteristic halo. Treatment is with amphotericin B and fluconazole.

6. Coccidiodomycosis—caused by *C. immitis* from the soil of the **southwest United States**, especially in California (the San Joaquin Valley) and in Arizona. The CNS is involved in $<33\%$ of cases with meningitis or cerebritis with granulomas. There are large sporangia filled with endospores. Treatment is with intrathecal amphotericin B and the mortality is 50%.

7. Aspergillosis—caused by *A. fumigatus* or *A. flavus* from the soil. It is the third most frequent fungal CNS infection. It is named from its sporangia that resembles a container of holy water

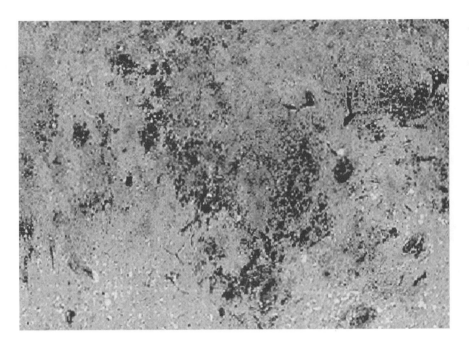

Figure 30   Aspergillus encephalitis (H and E); hemorrhagic cerebritis with branching septate hyphae.

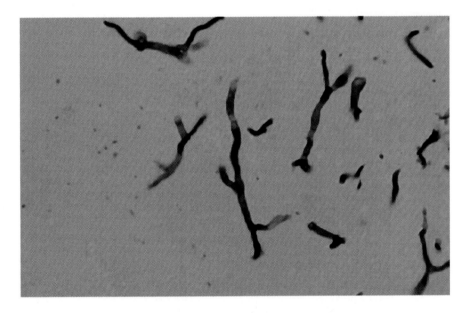

Figure 31   Aspergillus (silver stain); branching septate hyphae.

and only forms when growing with contact to air. It is rarely diagnosed before death. It is **angioinvasive** causing hemorrhagic cerebritis and rarely meningitis. It has branching septate hyphae. Treatment is with amphotericin B and 5-fluorocytosine (**Figs. 30 and 31**).

8. Mucormycosis—the fungus is from the soil. Rhinocerebral involvement is most common in **diabetic patients with acidosis** or dehydrated children with diarrhea and **immunosuppression** who develop acidosis. It causes periorbital swelling, proptosis, and nasal discharge. It spreads by direct extension from the sinuses through the veins to the orbit, cavernous sinus,

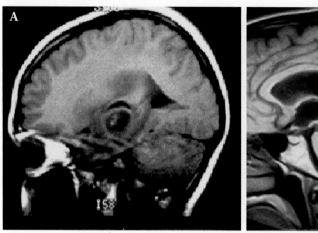
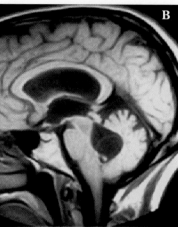

Figure 32   Cysticercosis. Noninfused sagittal T1-weighted MRIs demonstrate cystic lesions with a scolex in the left temporal lobe (A) and in the fourth ventricle (B).

and the brain. There is also spread from the lungs. It is angioinvasive causing deep **hemorrhagic necrosis** and ischemic strokes. It has nonseptate **right-angle branching hyphae**. Treatment is with amphotericin B.

F.   Parasites

1.   Nematodes (roundworms)

(a)   Trichinosis—caused by *Trichinella spiralis*. There are <100 cases per year in the United States. It is obtained by ingestion of **undercooked pork** that contains infectious cysts. Lesions occur mainly in the skeletal muscle, but occasionally in the CNS causing meningitis. Treatment is with thiobendazole and steroids.

(b)   Angiostrongylus cantonensis—a rat lung worm that involves the CNS causing eosinophilic meningitis.

(c)   Strongyloidiasis—this worm can carry bacteria with it to the CNS and cause mixed meningitis.

2.   Platyhelminth (flatworms)

(a)   Cestodes (tapeworms)

(1)   Cysticercosis—caused by ***Taenia solium*, the pork tapeworm**. It is the **most frequent CNS parasitic disease** in the world. The human is the definitive host of the adult worm. Cysticercosis occurs when a human serves as the intermediate host and the cysticerci accumulate in the subcutaneous tissue, skeletal muscles, eyes, and central nervous system. It may cause meningitis, a parenchymal abscess, or an intraventricular abscess. Taeniasis (tapeworm infection) is contracted by ingestion of undercooked pork, whereas cysticercosis is contracted by ingestion of food with fecal contamination. Treatment is with praziquantel or albendazole (**Figs. 32 through 34**).

(2)   Echinococcus (**hydatid disease**)—caused by *E. granulosa*, a dog tapeworm. The intermediate host is sheep. Each cyst contains multiple larvae (**hydatid sand**), and rupture can lead to further cyst formation. Cysts form in the liver (65%), lung (20%), and brain (2%). Treatment is with mebendazole.

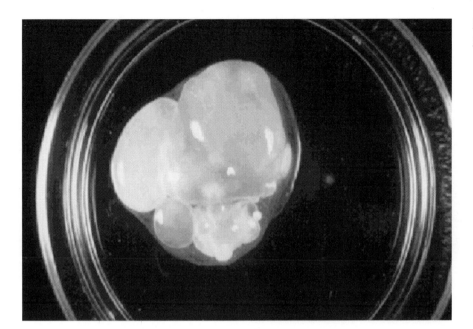

Figure 33   Cysticercosis (gross); cyst with larva.

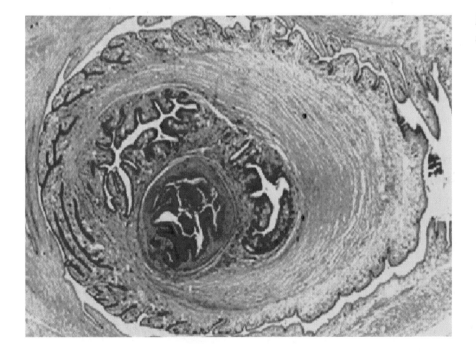

Figure 34   Cysticercosis (H and E); encysted larva with scolex.

(b) Trematodes (flukes)

(1) Schistosomiasis—caused by *S. haematobium* and *S. mansoni* which can infect the spinal cord, and by *S. japonicum*, which can infect the brain. They live in **blood vessels**, and the snail is the intermediate host. Treatment is with praziquantel.

(2) Paragonimiasis—caused by a fluke that resides in the lung and rarely enters the brain (1%) by way of the basal foramina. It can be acquired by ingestion of raw fish.

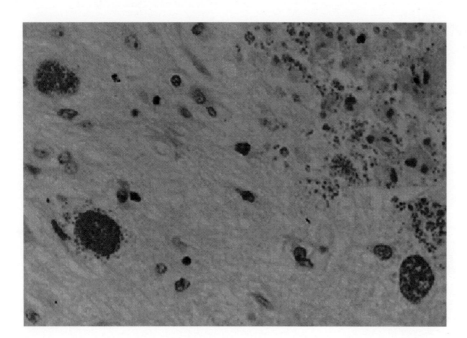

Figure 35   Toxoplasma (H and E); pseudocysts and multiple free tachyzoites.

G. Protozoa

1. Toxoplasmosis—caused by *T. gondii*, an **obligate intracellular** organism. The definitive host is the **cat**. Human infection is caused by ingestion of cat feces or raw meat. Serum antibodies are seen in 30% of the normal population. The cyst may lie dormant until the host becomes immunocompromised. It is the most frequent mass lesion in the brain in patients with AIDS. The **cyst** is full of and is surrounded by free **tachyzoites** that can be seen on H & E stain. Infection of the mother during pregnancy causes **congenital lesions** such as brain necrosis, periventricular calcification, hydrocephalus, hydranencephaly, chorioretinitis, and hepatosplenomegaly. Acquired infection may cause meningoencephalitis or abscesses. Treatment is with 4 weeks of **sulfadiazine and pyrimethamine** with leukovorin (to rescue the cells from the antifolate effects) or for the remainder of life in AIDS patients (**Fig. 35**).

2. Amoebic meningoencephalitis—caused by (1) *Naegleria fowler* from **freshwater ponds** or lakes that enters the skull through the cribriform plate and causes **basilar hemorrhagic meningitis** that may be rapidly fatal, (2) *Acanthamoeba* from contact lenses that gets in the corneal stroma (treatment may require a corneal transplant), and (3) *Entamoeba histolytica* that also may cause meningoencephalitis.

3. Malaria—caused mainly by ***Plasmodium falciparum***, but also by *Plasmodium vivax, Plasmodium malariae*, and *Plasmodium ovale*. One to 10% of cases involve the CNS and manifest as acute encephalopathy, fever, decreased mental status, seizures, and focal deficits. Symptoms may be due to cerebral hypoxia from **capillary obstruction** by infected red blood cells (RBCs).

4. Trypanosomiasis—caused by (1) ***T. brucei*** that causes **African sleeping sickness**, a meningoencephalitis transmitted by the **tsetse fly**, (2) *T. rhodesiense* that causes a more severe meningoencephalitis, (3) ***T. gambiense*** that is more chronic, and (4) ***T. cruzi*** that causes **Chagas's**

disease of South America that is transmitted by the **reduviid bug** and causes cardiomyopathy, megacolon, and congenital CNS lesions in children.

H. Viruses

1. Viruses—obligate intracellular parasites that depend on the host cell for protein synthesis and energy. They may contain either DNA or RNA. They have no organelles or nucleus and are not cells. They are surrounded by a capsid with protein subunits (capsomeres).

2. Neurotropic RNA viruses—picornavirus (poliomyelitis), togavirus (eastern and western equine encephalopathy and rubella), flavivirus (St. Louis encephalopathy), paramyxovirus (measles, SSPE), rhabdovirus (rabies), arena (lymphocytic choriomeningitis), bunyavirus (California group encephalitis), and retrovirus (HIV).

3. Neurotropic DNA viruses—papovavirus (PML) and the herpes group with HSV1 and 2, varicella-zoster, and CMV.

4. Infection transmission

    (a) Respiratory route—measles, mumps, and varicella-zoster.

    (b) GI route—poliovirus.

    (c) Subcutneous innoculation—rabies and arbovirus.

5. Virus access to the CNS

    (a) Blood—poliovirus.

    (b) Peripheral nerves—rabies.

6. DNA viruses

    (a) Circular without envelope—papovavirus JC and SV40.

    (b) Circular with envelope—Poxvirus.

    (c) Linear without envelope—adenovirus.

    (d) Linear with envelope—herpesvirus.

7. RNA viruses

    (a) Single strand, with sense, without envelope—picornavirus (poliovirus, echovirus, and coxsackievirus).

    (b) Single strand, with sense, with envelope—togavirus (rubella and eastern, western, and Venezuelan equine encephalopathies), retrovirus (HIV), and flavivirus (St. Louis and Japanese encephalopathies).

    (c) Single-strand, without sense, with envelope—paramyxovirus (measles, SSPE, mumps), rhabdovirus (rabies), bunyavirus (California encephalopathy), orthomyxovirus (influenza), and arenavirus (lymphocytic choriomeningitis).

8. Virus detection—by in-situ hybridization with radioactive complementary DNA or RNA or by polymerase chain reaction (PCR) used to amplify their DNA segments. HSV is persistent so it can always be recovered. Varicella-zoster becomes latent so it is intermittently recovered.

9. Viral (aseptic) meningitis—70% are caused by **enterovirus** (picornavirus: polio, echovirus, coxsackievirus) and mumps. It is self-limited and usually lasts up to 1 week.

    (a) Symptoms—fever, headache, and nuchal rigidity. There are no features of encephalitis such as decreased mental status, seizures, or focal deficits.

    (b) CSF evaluation—lymphocytic pleocytosis, normal protein and glucose (except decreased glucose with mumps and lymphocytic choriomeningitis virus in rodent handlers), and no bacteria or fungus on culture.

    (c) Epidemiology—it is most common in August and September. Nonviral aseptic meningitis may be caused by an adjacent sinus or mastoid bacterial infection, syphilis, *Cryptococcus*, TB, *Borrelia*, leukemia, lymphoma, and Behçet's disease.

10. Viral encephalitis—the most frequent **epidemic cause is arbovirus** and the most frequent **sporadic cause is HSV1**. In immunocompromised patients the most common viruses are HIV, CMV, and papovavirus (there are also infections from *Toxoplasma*, *Aspergillus*, and *Listeria*). Symptoms include seizures, decreased mental status, and focal deficits. There is a 5 to 20% mortality (HSV has 50% mortality) and 20% incidence of permanent sequelae.

11. Arboviruses—"Arthropod borne" by mosquitoes, ticks, etc. Reservoirs are birds, small mammals, and horses. Humans are dead-end hosts. They include togavirus, flavivirus, bunyavirus, and reovirus.

    (a) Eastern encephalopathy—the most severe and occurs in late summer in the eastern U.S. seaboard and has a 70% mortality.

    (b) Western encephalopathy—milder and occurs on the west coast of Canada, the United States, and Central America.

    (c) Venezuelan equine encephalopathy—mild, occurs in Central and South America, and has < 1% mortality.

    (d) LaCrosse encephalitis—the second most frequent encephalitis in the United States after enterovirus, has a low mortality, and occurs in the Midwest and New York.

    (e) St. Louis encephalitis—transmitted by birds and occurs in the summer in the Midwest and South.

    (f) Japanese encephalitis—the most frequent epidemic encephalitis in the world and has a 50% mortality.

    (g) Pathologic findings of all these viruses—demonstrates perivascular mononuclear infiltrates.

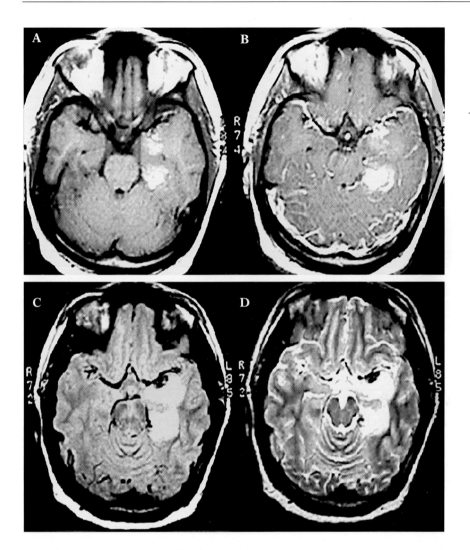

Figure 36   Herpes encephalitis. Axial MRI images demonstrate hemorrhagic and edematous left medial temporal lobe lesion: (A) noninfused T1-weighted, (B) infused T1-weighted, (C) proton density, and (D) T2-weighted MRI images.

12. Herpes encephalitis.

   (a) Herpes simplex virus (HSV)—enters through the eye, mouth, and genitals and reaches the CNS by the peripheral nerves. In the CNS, it remains relatively shielded from the host's immune system.

   (i)   The virus may travel from the skin to the olfactory nerve, trigeminal nerve, or to the trigeminal ganglion. It rarely spreads hematogenously. It is found in the trigeminal ganglion in 50% of normal adults and reactivates after trauma or immunosuppression.

   (ii) Findings—aseptic meningitis, encephalitis, myelitis, keratitis, skin lesions, and **hemorrhagic** necrosis of the **basal frontal and medial temporal lobes (Fig. 36)**.

   (iii) It is generally held that in children, the virus reaches the CNS by means of the olfactory mucosa and in adults by means of the trigeminal ganglion to the middle fossa. HSV1 is the most frequent cause of sporadic encephalitis.

   (iv) It usually affects those older than neonates, frequently involves limbic structures, and sequentially becomes bilateral. **HSV2 encephalitis affects mainly neonates and is more diffuse**.

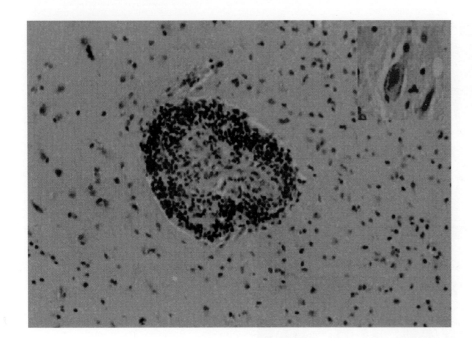

Figure 37   HSV-1 encephaliitis (H and E); lymphocytic perivascular cuffing. Inset with Cowdry A eosinophilic intranuclear inclusions.

(v) Diagnosis—by PCR to detect viral nucleic acid in the CSF (must be in first few days) or biopsy and culture of the anterior inferior temporal gyrus.

(vi) Pathologic examination (**Fig. 37**)—demonstrates **Cowdry type A inclusions** (intranuclear eosinophilic masses with a surrounding halo found in neurons, oligo-dendrocytes, and astrocytes). These inclusions are best seen in the first few days of the infection. The CSF culture is usually negative. Mortality is 50 to 60%. Treatment is with steroids and acyclovir IV for 14 days.

(b) Cytomegalovirus (CMV)—the largest herpesvirus. It is commonly found in all body fluids. It also produces Cowdry type A and intracytoplasmic inclusions. Diagnosis is by culture and in-situ hybridization. Intrauterine infections cause congenital malformations such as microcephaly, hydrocephalus, chorioretinitis, and microphthalmos (**Fig. 38**).

(c) Varicella zoster—the primary infection is varicella after which the virus becomes latent in the DRG. A reactivation is zoster (**shingles**) that mainly affects the elderly and immunocompromised. Two-thirds of cases are levels **T5-9**, and 15% of cases involve CN **V1** (trigeminal ophthalmic branch).

(i) Herpes infection of the geniculate ganglion (**Ramsey Hunt syndrome**)—may cause dysfunction of CN VII and VIII. It may lead to encephalitis, myelitis, or angiitis.

(ii) Pathologic examination—demonstrates intranuclear inclusions in the DRG and also the posterior horn gray matter, posterior roots, and meninges.

(iii) Treatment—skin lotions (calamine), capsaicin, acyclovir (must be given within 48 hours of rash formation to decrease the duration of disease, use 7-day oral course or 10-day IV course for immunocompromised patients or if > three dermatomes involved), and topical acyclovir for the eye with a V1 infection. Postherpetic pain is treated (although it responds poorly) with amitriptylin (Elavil), carbomazepine (Tegretol), and time.

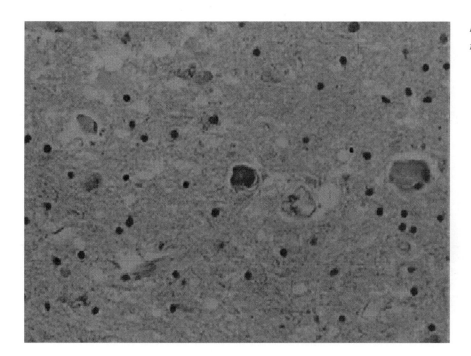

Figure 38   CMV (H and E); eosinophilic intranuclear and intracytoplasmic inclusions.

13. Rabies—acquired from the bites of skunks, foxes, coyotes, and bats. It may also be transmitted by aerosolized vectors inside caves where bats live. The virus travels through the **peripheral nerves** to the CNS and has an incubation period of 1 to 3 months.

   (a) The prodrome phase is followed by either a paralytic (Guillain-Barré–like) form or encephalitic (more frequent) form that progresses to coma and death 2 to 25 days after the onset of symptoms.

   (b) The virus destroys mainly **limbic neurons**. **Negri bodies** (intracytoplasmic eosinophyilic collections of ribonucleoproteins) are seen in 80% of cases and are especially prominent in the cerebellum (**Purkinjes cells**), brain stem, and hippocampus (**Fig. 39**).

   (c) Symptoms—include anxiety, dysphagia, and spasms of the throat when attempting to swallow (hydrophobia).

   (d) Treatment—by washing the wound with soap, water, and benzyl ammonium chloride (inactivates virus) and watching the biting animal for 10 days. If it becomes symptomatic, it should be sacrificed and the brain examined. If there are signs of rabies, treat with rabies immune globulin to provide 10 to 20 days of passive immunization. If one is at high risk, consider a vaccine.

14. Enteroviruses (poliovirus, coxsackievirus, and echoviruses; the human GI tract is the reservoir)

   (a) Poliovirus: (an ssRNA virus)

      (i) There are < 10 cases/year in the United States, and they are mostly vaccine related. Incubation is 7 to 21 days. Ten percent of cases develop viremia.

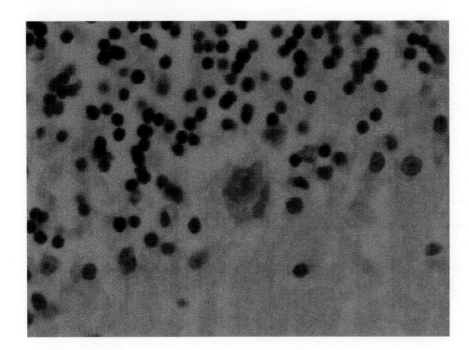

Figure 39   Rabies (H and E). Large intracytoplasmic eosinophilic Negri body in Purkinje's cell between the granular and molecular layers.

(ii)   Most infections are subclinical (nonparalytic form). The CNS is involved in 0.1 to 1% of cases with aseptic meningitis, encephalitis, and paralysis.

(iii)   **Anterior horn cells**—the most susceptible because they have increased numbers of viral receptors on their surface. The virus may also infect **Betz's cells** and **brain stem nuclei** (10 to 35% of patients develop bulbar palsy).

(iv)   Pathologic examination reveals perivascular mononuclear infiltrates and neuronophagia. There is no virus detected in the CSF (**Fig. 256**).

(v)   The risk of paralytic disease with the live attenuated oral vaccine is 1 in 2.5 million.

(vi)   Mortality is 5 to 10%. Motor strength usually returns in 4 months.

(b) Coxsackievirus and echoviruses—cause meningoencephalitis and polymyositis. They may be cultured from the CSF. The incidence is increased in patients with humoral immunity deficiencies.

15. Mumps—10% of the patients with mumps parotiditis develop meningitis. Before the routine use of the mumps vaccine, it accounted for 25% of viral encephalitis cases. It can be cultured from the CSF.

16. Measles—a postinfectious encephalomyelitis develops after the rash in 1 in 1000 cases. It is immune mediated and not directly caused by the virus.

(a) Subacute sclerosing pan encephalitis (**SSPE**)—occurs in children and adolescents (ages 5 to 15 years) after a measles infection that has usually occurred before 2 years of age.

(b) Chronic encephalitis develops with deteriorating school performance and behavioral changes followed by myoclonus, seizures, weakness, and death in 1 to 3 years.

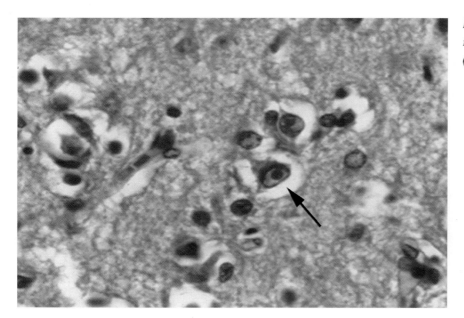

Figure 40   SSPE (H and E); eosinophilic intranuclear and intracytoplasmic inclusions (arrow).

(c) It affects both the **gray and white matter** with perivascular lymphocytes, neuronophagia, demyelination, and oligodendrocyte destruction.

(d) There are intranuclear and intracytoplasmic inclusions in the neurons and oligodendrocytes. The CSF has oligoclonal antibodies to the measles virus, no cells, and increased protein (**Fig. 40**).

(e) Diagnosis can be made by **periodic 2–3/s EEG spikes**, increased CSF Ig, and increased serum and CSF measles antibody titers.

17. Progressive multifocal leukoencephalopathy (PML)—from the **papovavirus** family that includes (1) the papillomavirus (associated with warts and cervical carcinoma), (2) the polyoma BK virus (associated with hemorrhagic cystitis), and (3) the **JC** and SV40 viruses (associated with PML).

(a) The **JC virus** normally resides in the kidney. PML occurs in immunocompromised people and is found in 2% of AIDS autopsies.

(b) Typically, CT and MRI demonstrate patchy hypodense white matter changes **without enhancement** or mass effect (**Fig. 41**).

(c) It is bilateral, asymmetric, subcortical, **spares the cortex**, and usually starts in the posterior centrum semiovale. There is **minimal cellular infiltration**, central destruction of oligodendrocytes and demyelination, and **peripheral swollen irregular oligodendrocytes** with ground-glass nuclei and intranuclear inclusions of "stick-and-ball" viral particles. CSF is normal (**Figs. 42 and 43**).

(d) Death occurs universally in a few months.

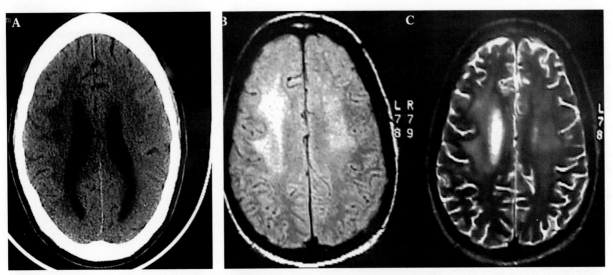

Figure 41   PML. CT (A), proton density (B), and T-2 weighted (C) MRIs demonstrating patchy white matter degeneration.

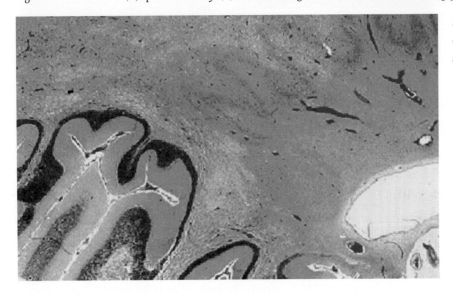

Figure 42   PML (H and E); low-power view demonstrates demyelination in cerebellar subcortical white matter.

18. Transmissible spongiform encephalitis—the incubation is months to years, but once deterioration is started it progresses rapidly to death. These are a heterogeneous collection of probable infections caused by SSPE, HIV, and prions.

19. Prions—these are not viruses because they are protein without nucleic acid. They are resistant to nucleases, ultraviolet light, and radiation. They can be inactivated with autoclaving, alkaline, 0.5% Na$^+$ hypochlorite, and 1% Na$^+$ dodecylsulfate.

   (a) A protease-resistant protein is coded on chromosome 20 and the production may be released by a DNA configuration change.

   (b) Prion diseases—kuru (in cannibals of New Guinea), scrappie (in sheep), possibly fatal familial insomnia, Creutzfeldt-Jakob disease (CJD), and Gerstmann-Straussler syndrome. CJD occurs in 50–65-year-old people and manifests as myoclonus, pyramidal and extrapyramidal degeneration, dementia, and visual deterioration.

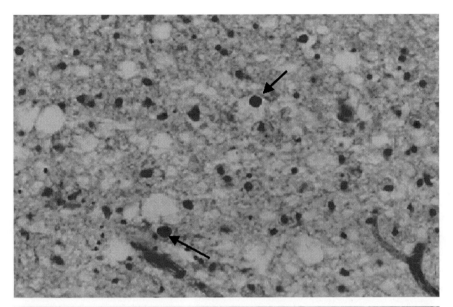

Figure 43   PML (H and E). High-power view demonstrates demyelination with surrounding enlarged bizarre oligodendrocyte nuclei (arrows).

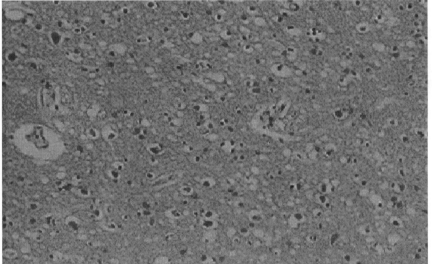

Figure 44   CJD (H and E); spongiform changes.

(c) There is a characteristic **EEG with bilateral sharp waves 1.5–2/s** that resemble PLEDS but are reactive to painful stimuli.

(d) CSF appears normal.

(e) Pathologic examination—demonstrates **spongiform changes** with astrocytosis but **no inflammation** most prominently in the cortex, putamen, and thalamus (**Fig. 44**). Five to 10% of patients have amyloid kuru plaques develop. Death occurs in less than 1 year.

(f) Gerstmann-Straussler syndrome—ataxia, dysarthria, hyporeflexia, and dementia, without myoclonus. Its transmission is both autosomal dominant and sporadic, and Kuru plaques are seen in the cerebellum. These diseases can be transmitted to laboratory animals that develop the same microscopic changes.

(g) Diagnosis can be made by immunostaining with protease-resistant protein antisera.

20.   Acquired immune deficiency syndrome (AIDS)

(a) Acquired immune deficiency syndrome (AIDS)—caused by a retrovirus that contains RNA. It requires reverse transcriptase to convert its RNA to DNA and allow replication.

(b) HTLV-1 (human T-cell lymphotropic virus)—causes a chronic myelopathy with spastic paresis but no sensory deficit and involves the anterior and lateral columns. It occurs mainly in the tropics (**tropical spastic paraparesis**) and Japan.

(c) HTLV-2—associated with chronic T-cell leukemia and lymphoma.

(d) HIV (HTLV3)—a lentivirus with a surface molecule that interacts with T4. It is associated with *Pneumocystis* infections and Kaposi's sarcoma. Viral latency is 8 years, and once AIDS ensues, 50% die in < 1 year and most in < 3 years. Fifty percent of cases have neurologic symptoms develop and 80% have CNS abnormalities. CNS complications at various stages include:

(i)   Seroconversion—aseptic meningitis, acute encephalitis, and myelopathy.

(ii)   HIV-positive—asymptomatic or AIDS related complex with aseptic meningitis.

(iii) AIDS—aseptic meningitis, AIDS dementia complex, lymphoma, and vacuolar myelopathy.

(e) AIDS dementia complex—**the most frequent AIDS disorder** seen in 50% of patients. It is believed to be caused by encephalitis or the viral impact on the neurons. It consists of a triad of cognitive dysfunction (subcortical dementia), behavioral changes (psychoses and hallucinations), and motor deficits (by centrum semiovale and brain stem involvement).

(f) Congenital lesions—atrophy, hydrocephalus ex-vacuo, microcephaly, facial dysmorphism, and basal ganglia calcifications.

(g) HIV encephalitis—pathologic examination demonstrates microglial nodules in the white matter and subcortical gray matter with focal demyelination, neuronal loss, reactive astrocytosis, and calcifications in the parenchymal blood vessels and basal ganglia. There are characteristic **multinucleated giant cells** that are unique to HIV in the CNS and are of macrophage origin (**Fig. 45**).

(h) **Vacuolar myelopathy**—mainly involves the **posterior and lateral columns** of the low **thoracic** levels. Pathologic examination demonstrates vacuolar changes with lipid-laden macrophages. It is detected in 50% of AIDS autopsies but less often clinically.

(i) Peripheral neuropathy—seen in 5–38% of AIDS cases and is caused by DDI chemotherapy, demyelination, and arteritis.

(j) Myopathy—seen in 20% of AIDS cases, is characterized by inflammation, atrophy, polymyositis, and AZT-induced mitochondrial changes.

(k) Toxoplasmosis—seen in 10% of autopsy cases. It is the most frequent cause of focal neurologic symptoms in AIDS. Toxoplasmosis may cause focal or diffuse lesions and predominantly causes basal ganglia and gray/white junction lesions. The serum IgG level is increased with infection and pathologic examination demonstrates a mononuclear inflammation with extracellular tachyzoites and encysted bradyzoites (**Fig. 35**). Treatment is with pyrimethamine and sulfadiazine for 14 days.

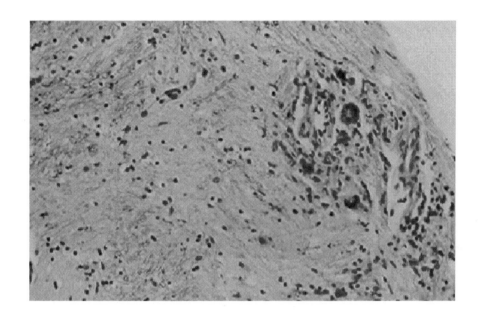

Figure 45   HIV encephalitis (LFB-H and E). Microglial nodule with characteristic multinucleated giant cells.

(l) CMV—seen in 30% of AIDS autopsies but only 10% are symptomatic with necrotizing encephalomyelitis. Pathologic examination demonstrates microglial nodules mainly in the gray matter and rarely in the white matter (unlike HIV). There are Cowdry type A intranuclear and intracytoplasmic inclusions in the neurons and astrocytes.

(m) PML—described previously.

(n) Primary CNS lymphoma—seen in 5% of autopsies. It is invariably of B-cell origin with large or mixed large/small cell types. They are usually periventricular with perivascular spread. EBV is frequently detected in the cells and may play a role in the development of the lymphoma.

(o) *Cryptococcus*—in the normal population it causes meningitis, whereas in immunocompromised patients it causes encephalitis and cryptococomas in the basal ganglia and midbrain.

(p) AIDS symptomatic infections—HIV encephalitis (60%), *Toxoplasma* (30%), *Cryptococcus* (5%), PML (4%), and less frequently lymphoma (not an infection), TB, syphilis, varicella-zoster, and CMV.

21. Rasmussen's chronic encephalitis—occurs in childhood and causes progressive deficits and seizures (classically complex partial status epilepticus) with unilateral atrophy. It may be caused by CMV infection or by antibodies to glutamate receptors.

22. Postinfectious encephalitis

(a) SSPE—see earlier discussion. It develops several years after a measles infection. There are increased neutralized measles virus Ig titers in the serum and CSF. Pathologic examination demonstrates atrophy, perivascular lymphocytosis, demyelination, and increased eosinophilic intranuclear and intracytoplasmic inclusions in the neurons and oligodendrocytes. It affects children and young adults and develops in 1 in 1,000,000 cases of measles. Findings are as described earlier. Death occurs within 1 to 3 years.

(b) Acute disseminated encephalomyelitis—immune-mediated disease that occurs after a **viral infection or a vaccination**.

      (i)   It most commonly occurs with varicella-zoster, measles, upper respiratory infection, rabies vaccination, diphtheria, smallpox, tetanus, typhoid, and influenza.

      (ii)   Pathologic examination demonstrates perivascular mononuclear infiltrates with a zone of demyelination along the course of the venules.

      (iii) All ages are affected, but it usually occurs in children and young adults.

      (iv) Symptoms occur 1 to 3 weeks after the infection. It follows a rapid course, although some patients survive.

      (v)   Treatment is with steroids. Mortality is 20 to 50%.

23. CSF glucose—low with fungal infections, TB, carcinomatous meningitis, and sarcoid.

24. IL-1—released in response to endotoxins and stimulates the interleukin cascade to increase T-cell proliferation.

25. TNF—stimulates IL-1 production and activates neutrophils.

I.   Congenital infections (TORCH)

A.   Congenital infections are acquired in one of three ways:

1.   Hematogenous spread through the placenta (*Toxoplasma* and viruses).

2.   Ascending from the cervix (bacteria).

3.   During passage through the birth canal (herpes, this mechanism causes neonatal rather than true congenital infection).

4.   They may cause developmental changes or tissue destruction. Larger organisms such as bacteria, fungus, and protozoa are unable to enter the embryo before 3 to 4 months, but viruses may pass through the placenta.

5.   The usual time frame for congenital infections is first trimester (rubella), 4 months (syphilis), 5 months (*Toxoplasma*), paranatal (bacteria, HIV), during passage through birth canal (HSV2, HIV).

B.   Cytomegalovirus (CMV)

1.   CMV is the **most frequent congenital CNS infection**.

2.   It causes migration disorders during the first or early second trimester. Transmission is transplacental. Seventy-five percent of women have serum CMV antibodies (which are protective), 1% of newborns have CMV detected in the urine and 10% of these have CNS infection.

3.   It affects the brain, heart, liver, and spleen. The virus has an affinity for the germinal matrix and causes perivascular necrosis and calcifications.

4.   Premature infants may have hepatosplenomegaly, jaundice, thrombocytopenia, chorioretinitis, seizures, mental retardation, optic atrophy, impaired hearing, and **hydrocephalus**.

5.   Diagnosis is made by cultures, immunoglobulin levels, and intracellular (intranuclear and intracytoplasmic) inclusions on biopsy specimens.

6.   Radiographs may demonstrate microcephaly and **periventricular eggshell calcifications**.

C. *Toxoplasma*

1. *Toxoplasma* is the second most frequent congenital CNS infection.

2. It occurs in 1 in 1000 to 1 in 10,000 pregnancies and is acquired by hematogenous spread through the placenta. There may be giant cell granulomas with atrophy of the basal ganglia, periventricular white matter, and cortex.

3. Unlike CMV, there are **no migrational disorders or periventricular calcifications**. The infection is significant if acquired before 26 weeks gestation.

4. Findings include seizures, microcephaly, and spontaneous abortions. There is a classical triad that includes **hydrocephalus**, bilateral **chorioretinitis**, and **cranial calcifications**. Deafness is the most common late manifestation.

5. Treat with spiramycin if the mother seroconverts in 2 to 3 months. If the mother seroconverts after 4 months, use pyrimethamine and sulfadiazine.

D. Rubella

1. Rubella is transmitted transplacentally.

2. The virus inhibits cell multiplication to cause an insufficient number of cells in the brain (less neurons, astrocytes, and oligodendrocytes) and also is teratogenic and destructive.

3. The infection may cause meningoencephalitis, vasculopathy with ischemia and necrosis, microcephaly, decreased myelin, and **cortical and basal ganglia calcifications**. If the infection occurs before 12 weeks, the effects are very severe and spontaneous abortion is likely. If it occurs after 12 weeks, the infection is less severe.

4. Congenital rubella syndrome occurs with infection in the first trimester and includes chorioretinitis, **cataracts**, glaucoma, microphthalmos, microcephaly, mental retardation, and **deafness**.

5. During infection, the CSF has increased mononuclear cells and IgMs. Prevent with maternal vaccination before pregnancy.

E. HSV

1. HSV is transmitted transvaginally.

2. It occurs in 1 in 200 to 1 in 5000 births. Eighty-five percent are caused by HSV2 and rare early lesions cause death, chorioretinitis, and microcephaly. The virus has a predilection for vascular endothelial cells and causes thrombosis and hemorrhagic stroke that develop 2 to 4 weeks postpartum.

3. Pathologic examination demonstrates microglial nodules and intranuclear inclusions. The infection is diffuse and causes white matter edema without the temporal localization.

4. The most frequent manifestation are skin, eye, and mouth lesions, but if no treatment is given, the infection may disseminate with an 80% mortality (only 50% with treatment).

5. The CNS is involved in 30% and produces fever, seizures, and lethargy. HSV1 affects older children.

F. HIV

1. HIV can be transmitted perinatally. Thirty percent of HIV–infected mothers transmit the virus to the children.

2. Pathologic examination demonstrates brain atrophy and basal ganglia calcifications.

3. Symptoms include weight loss, failure to thrive, diarrhea, and fever. Most die in 1 year.

G. Syphilis

    1. Syphilis has transplacental transmission at 4 to 7 months.

    2. Hutchinson's triad—dental disorders, bilateral **deafness**, and interstitial keratitis.

    3. The other symptoms of syphilis are the same as in adults, but occur much earlier at 9 to 15 years. Hydrocephalus and stroke may occur.

    4. The child should be treated with penicillin until the CSF is acellular and has a normal protein.

H. *Listeria*—causes increased abortions and premature deliveries.

I. Calcifications—caused mainly by CMV (periventricular) and *Toxoplasma* (disseminated).

J. Cardiac malformations—caused by rubella.

K. Deafness—caused by rubella and CMV.

VIII. ONCOLOGY

A. General Neuro-oncology

    1. Primary brain tumors are slightly more common than metastatic tumors. The most frequent is glioblastoma multiforme (GBM) followed by meningioma. Gliomas are more common in males and meningiomas are more common in females.

    2. Children—brain malignancies are the second most common cancer after leukemia. Seventy percent are infratentorial. The most frequent types are cerebellar astrocytoma (33%), brain stem glioma (25%), medulloblastoma (25%), and ependymoma (12%). Twenty percent of brain tumors occur before 15 years of age. The most frequent supratentorial tumors in children are low-grade astrocytomas (50%), craniopharyngiomas (12%), and optic gliomas (12%).

    3. Neonates and infants (<2 years)—brain tumors are rare and usually congenital. Two-thirds are supratentorial. The most common is **teratoma**, followed by PNET, **high-grade astrocytoma**, and choroid plexus papilloma. Findings include macrocephaly, hydrocephalus, split sutures, seizures, and focal deficits. Most of the tumors are highly malignant and have a poor prognosis.

    4. Older children—most brain tumors are infratentorial. The most common types are astrocytoma (50%), PNET (15%), craniopharyngioma (10%), ependymoma (10%), and pineal tumor (3%).

    5. Adults—primary tumors are slightly more commmon than metastatic tumors in clinical series. Seventy percent are supratentorial. The most frequent tumors are GBM, metastatic tumors, anaplastic astrocytoma, meningioma, pituitary tumors, and vestibular schwanomas. The most frequent infratentorial tumors are metastases, schwanoma, meningioma, epidermoid, hemangioblastoma (the most frequent primary intra-axial posterior fossa tumor), and brain stem glioma.

    6. In the spinal cord—the most frequent epidural lesions are metastatic. The most frequent intradural/extramedullary lesions are schwannoma and meningioma. The most frequent intramedullary lesions are astrocytoma and ependymoma.

7. Causes of tumors

   (a) Radiation—associated with meningiomas, fibrosarcomas, and gliomas.

   (b) Immunosuppression—associated with lymphomas.

   (c) Viruses—The Epstein Barr virus is associated with Burkitt's lymphoma and nasopharyngeal carcinoma and the human papillomavirus is associated with cervical carcinoma.

   (d) Chemotherapy—by nitrosurea.

   (e) Genetics—as seen in phakomatoses and Turcot's syndrome.

8. Prognosis of gliomas depends on: (1) age, (2) histologic findings (especially necrosis), (3) Karnofsky score, (4) neurologic deficit, and (5) extent of resection.

9. Analysis of tumors—light microscopy, electron microscopy, immunohistochemistry, and in situ mRNA hybridization.

10. Immunohistochemical stains

   (a) Alfa-feto protein (AFP)—embryonal carcinoma, endodermal sinus tumor.

   (b) Chromogranin—pituitary adenoma.

   (c) Common leukocyte antigen—lymphoma, germinoma.

   (d) Cytokeratin—carcinoma, craniopharyngioma, chordoma.

   (e) Desmin—rhabdosarcoma, teratoma.

   (f) Epithelial membrane antigen—carcinoma, meningioma, epithelial cysts.

   (g) Glial fibrillary acidic protein (**GFAP**)—astrocytomas, other glial tumors.

   (h) HMB 45—Melanoma.

   (i) βHCG—Choriocarcinoma.

   (j) Immunoglobulins k and l chains—lymphomas.

   (k) Neurofilament and synaptophysin—ganglioglioma, PNET.

   (l) Pituitary hormones—pituitary adenoma.

   (m) PSA—prostate carcinoma.

   (n) S100—schwannoma, neurofibroma, glioma, PNET, chordoma, melanoma, and renal cell carcinoma.

   (o) **Synaptophysin**—tumors with neurons (ganglioglioma, central neurocytoma, etc.)

   (p) Transthyretin—choroid plexus tumors.

   (q) **Vimentin**—meningioma.

   (r) Many tumors have unexpected overlaps.

11. Assessment of proliferative capacity

    (a) G1 phase—preparation for DNA synthesis (**susceptible to radiation**).

    (b) S phase—DNA synthesis (resistant to radiation).

    (c) G2 phase—preparation for mitosis.

    (d) M phase—mitosis (**susceptible to radiation**).

    (e) G0 phase—normal cell activity phase.

Only a small portion of the dividing cells are in the M phase, so the mitotic index is misleading. Flow cytometry is more accurate because it stains DNA and counts the number of cells with double DNA. Also available are cytophotometry, DNA synthesis markers, and proliferation antigens that appear during the cell cycle (Ki67 is in all stages except G0).

12. Oncogenes

    (a) Oncogene—expression of this gene can cause the cell to enter an unrestrained replication cycle (malignant change). They may be introduced by a virus. Examples are *c-myc* oncogene (activation causes Burkitt's lymphoma) and *n-myc* oncogene 9 (activation causes neuroblastoma).

    (b) Proto-oncogene—a gene locus that becomes an oncogene by deletion or translocation.

    (c) Tumor supressor gene—a gene in the normal genome that when lost or mutated allows malignant growth to occur. Tumor supressor gene loss is associated with gliomas (chromosomes 9, 10, and 17), meningiomas (chromosome 22), and retinoblastomas (chromosome 13). The **p53 nuclear protein gene** is a tumor supressor gene on **chromosome 17p** and alterations are seen in 33% of astrocytomas.

13. Paraneoplastic syndromes (possibly autoimmune or viral)

    (a) Limbic encephalitis—subacute encephalitis. Gross examination appears normal. There are perivascular mononuclear infiltrates but no viral inclusions. The **medial temporal lobes**, cingulate gyrus, and insula are predominantly affected. There are usually bilateral hyperintense lesions on T2-weighted MRI. It is most common in men in their mid-60s and manifests as memory impairment and altered mental status. It is associated with **small cell lung carcinoma**. Limbic encephalitis should be differentiated from herpes encephalitis.

    (b) **Anti-Yo antibodies**—cause cerebellar degeneration and are associated with ovarian and breast cancer.

    (c) **Anti-Hu antibodies**—cause sensory neuropathy and are associated with oat cell pulmonary carcinoma or lymphoma.

    (d) Anti-Ri antibodies—cause opsoclonus and are associated with breast cancer.

    (e) Eaton-Lambert syndrome—antibodies to the presynaptic voltage-gated Ca^{++} channels; associated with oat cell lung carcinoma. See section XXXI.

    (f) Stiffman syndrome—involuntary muscle spasms and rigidity; 60% have antibodies to glutamic acid decarboxylase.

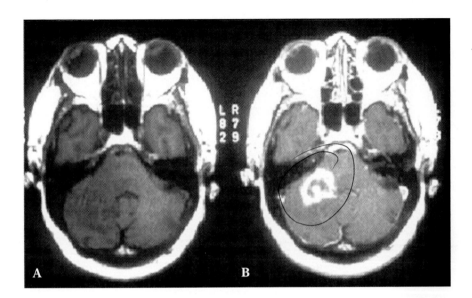

Figure 46   Radiation necrosis. Noninfused (A) and infused (B) axial T1-weighted MRIs demonstrate the irregularly enhancing low-density lesion.

14. Radiation

(a) Radiation-sensitive tumors—**lymphoma and germ cell tumors** (mainly germinoma but to some extent the others) are very radiosensitive. Meningioma, pineal tumors, craniopharyngioma, pituitary tumors, vestibular schwannoma, and metastatic tumors are less sensitive.

(b) Standard radiation doses.

    (i)   Metastatic tumors—**30 Gy over 2 weeks**.

    (ii) Gliomas—**6000 cGy in 200 cGy daily fractions**.

    (iii) Doses higher than these are much more likely to cause radiation necrosis.

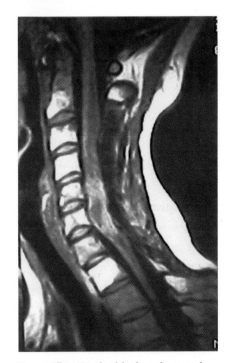

Figure 47   Vertebral body radiation changes. Sagittal T1-weighted MRI demonstrates the high-signal intensity changes in the vertebral bodies because of increased fat content.

(c) Radiation necrosis—white matter coagulation necrosis or demyelination caused by vessels with hyalin intimal thickening with fibrinoid necrosis and thrombosis. The neurons are relatively resistant. Symptoms usually start 3 months to 3 years (average **18 months**) after radiation. Radiation myelopathy is reduced if the daily fraction is kept less than 200 cGy, the weekly fraction less then 900 cGy, and the total dose less then 6000 cGy. Symptoms begin with paresthesias/dysesthesias in the hands or feet and Lhermitte's sign. There is no local pain, and it may progress irregularly. T2-weighted MRI demonstrates increased signal intensity and pathologic examination demonstates necrosis of the gray and white matter. Treatment is with steroids (**Figs. 46 and 47**).

(d) Radiation may induce tumor formation such as sarcomas, GBMs, and meningiomas.

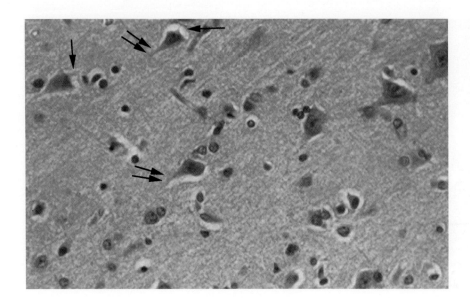

Figure 48   Normal gray matter (H and E). Neurons oriented with large apical dendrites (double arrows) toward the pia and axons (arrows) toward the ventricles.

B. Glial tumors

1. Astrocyte types are (1) fibrillary—more numerous, mainly in the white matter, stains with PTAH, silver, and GFAP; (2) protoplasmic—mainly in the gray matter and has a larger nucleus but less cytoplasm; and (3) gemistocytic—swollen active astrocyte with increased fibers and cytoplasm and appears often with injury, stroke, toxin, infection, or tumor.

2. Circumscribed astrocytic tumors—low grade, good prognosis, and frequently cystic.

(a) Juvenile pilocytic astrocytoma (JPA)—the second most common pediatric brain tumor. It accounts for one-third of pediatric gliomas and 5 to 10% of all gliomas. It is most frequently located in the cerebellum, brain stem, optic pathway, and infundibulum. In adults it is more common near the third ventricle. The peak age is 10 years. Sixty percent are cystic, and they usually have a mural red-tan nodule. There is a **biphasic pattern** of loose cells and microcysts and also dense elongated hairlike astrocytes with **Rosenthal fibers**. They tend to be noncystic in the medulla and optic pathway. Leptomeningeal invasion, nuclear atypia, multinucleated cells, and vascular proliferation are frequently noted but are not adverse prognostic indicators. Approximately 10% contain calcium. The nodule may enhance. There is usually no necrosis. Survival is 86 to 100% at 5 years, 83% at 10 years, and 70% at 20 years (**Figs. 48 through 52**).

(b) Pleomorphic xantho astrocytoma (PXA)—the peak age is 7 to 25 years. Seizures are frequent. There is a **temporal lobe** predominance. They are usually superficial and involve the **cortex** and leptomeninges but not the dura. They tend to be **cystic with a mural nodule**. Pathologic examination demonstrates **bizarre pleomorphic astrocytes** with **xanthomatous fat cells**, spindle cells, and multinucleated cells. There are frequent mitoses, calcifications, a rich reticulin network, and no necrosis. They have a good prognosis, and most patients are alive at 17 years. There have been occasional reported transformations to GBM.

(c) Subependymal giant cell astrocytoma—the peak age is < 20 years. Symptoms are by hydrocephalus and seizures. They are located near the **foramen of Monro**. They

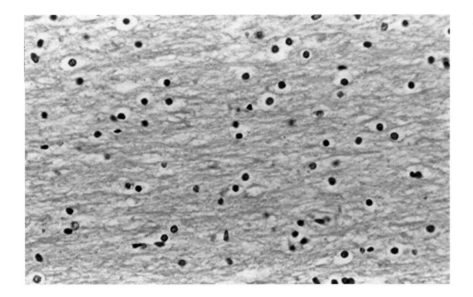

Figure 49   Normal white matter (H and E). Normal oligodendrocytes interspersed in a fibrillary backround.

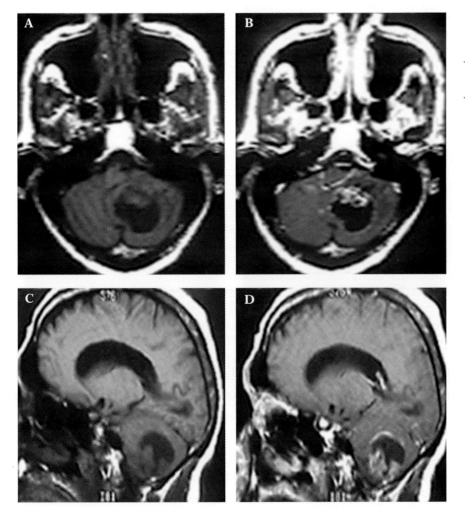

Figure 50   Juvenile pilocytic astrocytoma. Axial T1-weighted MRI (A) noninfused and (B) infused, and sagittal T1-weighted (C) noninfused and (D) infused MRIs with enhancing nodule in cerebellar cystic lesion.

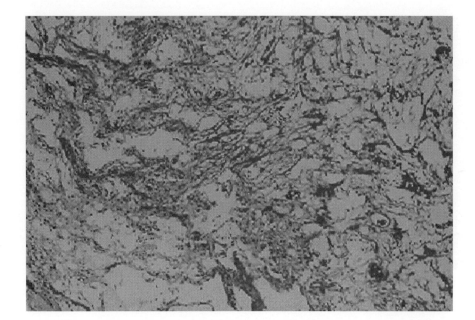

Figure 51   Pilocytic astrocytoma (H and E). Biphasic histologic specimens of loose microcystic components and dense components with prominent eosinophilic granular bodies.

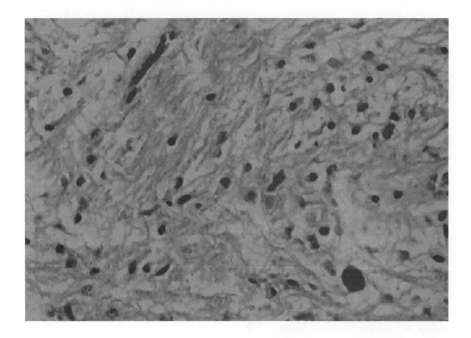

Figure 52   Pilocytic astrocytoma (H and E); eosinophilic Rosenthal fibers.

enhance, have frequent **calcifications**, may be cystic and lobulated, and tend to be well demarcated. Pathologic examination reveals **large multinucleated cells** and rare mitoses. These tumors are seen in 15% of tuberous sclerosis (**TS**) cases, and if it forms without a diagnosis of TS, it is considered a forme-fruste (**Figs. 53 and 54**).

3. Diffuse astrocytic tumors—infiltrative and carry a worse prognosis. They may be fibrillary (most frequent), protoplasmic, gemistocytic (probably a worse prognosis if > 20% of cells are gemistocytic), or mixed. The grade is determined by the degree of anaplasia with increased cel-

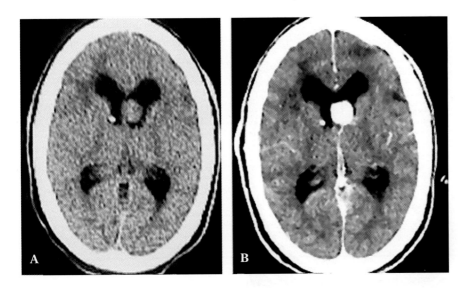

Figure 53   Subependymal giant cell astrocytoma. Axial noninfused (A) and infused (B) CTs demonstrating a large enhancing mass in the lateral ventricle. Also noted is a calcified tuber on the right lateral ventricular wall.

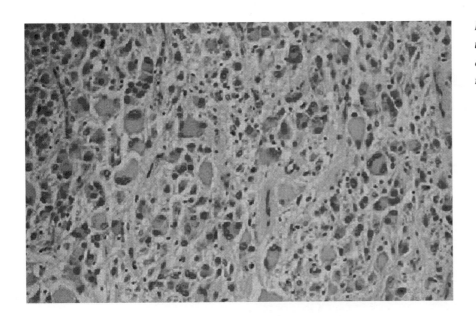

Figure 54   Subependymal giant cell astrocytoma (H and E). Enlarged cells with abundant eosinophilic cytoplasm and large nuclei with prominent central nucleoli.

lularity, nuclear pleomorphism, mitoses, endothelial proliferation, necrosis, and to a lesser extent, pseudopallisading features.

(a) Grades 1 and 2 (low grade astrocytoma)—well differentiated, comprise 15% of astrocytomas, peak age 30 years, **male predominance**, most frequently in the **frontal white matter**, and most commonly **fibrillary**. They tend to be hypodense, minimally enhancing, and occasionally cystic. Pathologic examination reveals a gray-colored homogenous tumor with indistinct borders that expands the white matter. There are no mitoses and only rarely hemorrhage or edema. 15% calcify. It is differentiated from reactive gliosis because it is **patternless**, violates the gray/white junction, has microcysts, **microcalcifications**, and increased nuclear atypia and pleomorphism. The

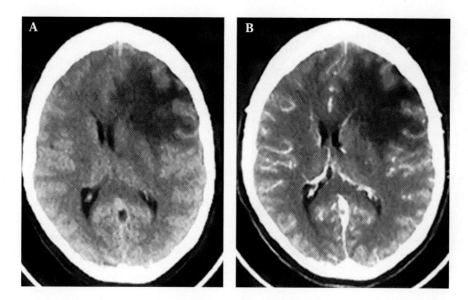

Figure 55   Low-grade astrocytoma. Axial CT (A) noninfused and (B) infused with nonenhancing left frontal hypodense mass.

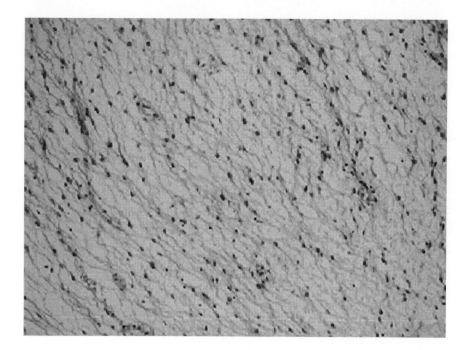

Figure 56   Fibrillary (grade 2) astrocytoma (H and E). Patternless but uniform infiltrating cells.

5-year survival with total resection and radiation is 70% and with subtotal resection and radiation is 38%. Median survival is 8.2 years and 50% increase in grade over time (**Figs. 55 and 56**).

(b) Grade 3 (anaplastic astrocytoma, AA)—comprise 30% of astrocytomas, peak age is 40 to 60 years, with **male predominance**. CT reveals a mixed density lesion with irregular rim enhancement and edema. Pathologic examination demonstrates increased cellularity, nuclear atypia, mitotic figures, with or without endothelial hyperplasia, and no necrosis. There may be hemorrhages or cysts and **rarely calcification**. There are frequent gemistocytes (>20/HPF denotes worse prognosis). They spread through white matter tracts, and there is frequent ependymal and CSF dissemination. **Secondary**

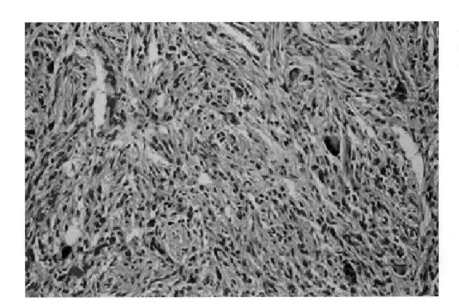

Figure 57   Anaplastic (grade 3) astrocytoma (H and E). Increased cellularity with hyperchromatic pleomorphic nuclei.

structures of Scherer are located around neurons in the gray matter, the subpial region, and the subependymal zone. The median survival is 2 to 3 years (**Fig. 57**).

(c) Grade 4 glioblastoma multiforme (GBM)—comprise 50% of astrocytomas, the **most frequent primary brain tumor** (20%), peak age is 45 to 60 years, with **male predominance**. GBM and AA are among the four most common tumors in children < 2 years old.

   (i)   The location is most commonly **deep frontotemporal**. CT reveals a **heterogeneous lesion** that is cystic in 85% of cases with **rare calcifications**. Angiogram demonstrates a vascular mass with arteriovenous shunting and early draining veins (**Figs. 58**).

   (ii) Pathologic examination is heterogeneous with cysts, degeneration, **necrosis**, hemorrhages, edema, marked hypercellularity, nuclear atypia, frequent mitoses, **pseudopallisading**, and **endovascular hyperplasia** with glomeruloid structures (**Figs. 59 and 60**).

   (iii) The tumor cells follow white matter tracts (especially the corpus callosum) and may invade dura, disseminate in the CSF, and rarely produce distant metastases. They are occasionally **multicentric** (3 to 6%). GBMs are associated with increased epithelial growth factor receptor (on chromosome 7). The median survival is 8 to 18 months.

   (iv) Giant cell GBM—has multinucleated giant cells, increased reticulin, and a slightly better prognosis probably because the giant cells can no longer divide. The small cell GBM has a worse prognosis.

   (v)   **Gliomatosis cerebri**—one or two diffusely enlarged hemispheres filled with tumor, or diffuse enlargement of the cerebellum or brain stem. It is most common at 20 to 30 years, and there are no focal masses (**Fig. 61**).

(d) Protoplasmic astrocytoma—small stellate cells with delicate processes that are predominantly in the gray matter. Prognosis is similar to fibrillary astrocytomas.

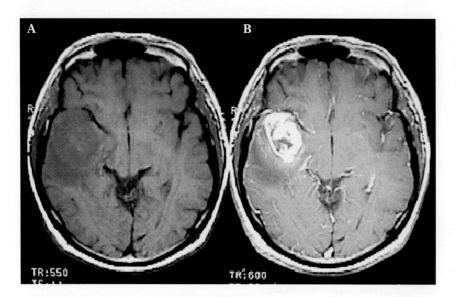

Figure 58   High-grade astrocytoma. Axial noninfused (A) and infused (B) T1-weighted MRIs demonstrating a temporal lesion with irregular cystic enhancement.

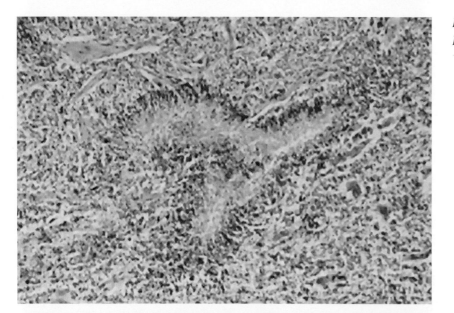

Figure 59   GBM (H and E); pseudopallisading necrosis.

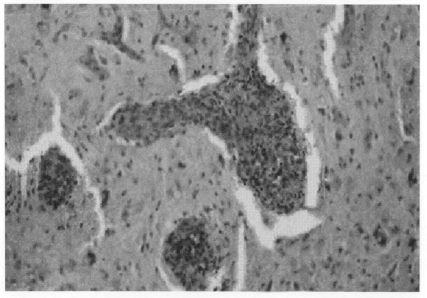

Figure 60   GBM (H and E); endothelial proliferation.

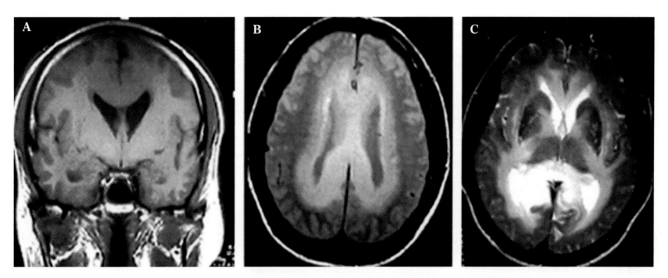

Figure 61   Gliomatosis cerebri. Coronal T1-weighted (A), axial proton density (B), and T2-weighted (C) MRIs demonstrating diffuse bilateral white matter infiltration by the tumor.

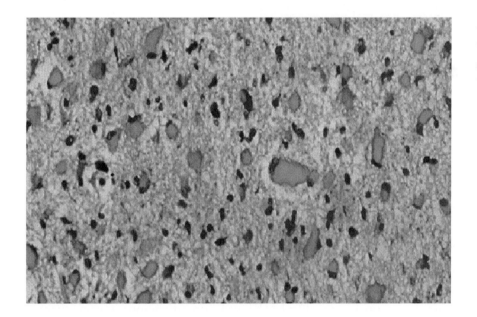

Figure 62   Gemistocytic astrocytoma (H and E). Enlarged astrocytes with prominent eosinophilic cytoplasm and eccentric nuclei.

(e) Adult pilocytic astrocytoma—unlike the juvenile variety. It is not circumscribed and has a worse prognosis.

(f) Gemistocytic astrocytoma—defined by > 20% gemistocytes, contains **large cells with eccentric eosinophyllic cytoplasm**, and has a **worse prognosis (Fig. 62)**.

(g) Gliosarcoma (Feigin tumor)—comprises 2% of GBMs, peak age is 40 to 60 years, and it most commonly involves the temporal lobe superficially with dural invasion. Lesions are firm, circumscribed, lobulated, and contain fascicles of spindle cell sarcoma with interspersed GBM cells. Silver stains the reticulin in the sarcoma component, and GFAP stains the GBM component. There are frequent intracranial and extracranial metastases (15 to 30%). It is postulated that the sarcoma arises from the vascular structures in the GBM or from leptomeningeal fibroblasts. The survival is similar to GBM.

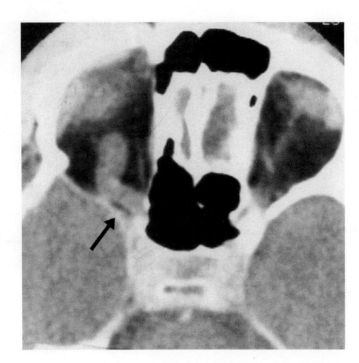

Figure 63   Optic glioma. Non-infused axial CT demonstrating thickened right optic nerve (arrow).

(h) Optic glioma—peak age is 3 to 5 years, **female** predominance, 20% may act malignantly, associated with **NF1**. Treatment is by: (1) if distal to the chiasm, remove optic nerve and attached globe; and (2) if the chiasm is involved, resect up to the chiasm preserving vision in the better eye and consider radiation if tumor progression is noted (**Figs. 63 through 65**).

(i) Brain stem glioma—accounts for 20% of intracranial tumors in children, usually **diffusely infiltrates** and enlarges the **pons**, progresses rapidly, and the 5-year survival is 30%. Symptoms begin with **cranial nerve palsies**, and hydrocephalus develops later. Treatment is with **radiation**. Biopsy is usually not necessary because the diffuse pontine lesion (hypointense on T1-weighted MRI and nonenhancing) is very characteristic. The prognosis is better with cystic lesions, dorsal exophytic lesions, and lesions involving the midbrain, medulla, or cervicomedullary junction. These lesions may be amenable to surgical resection (**Fig. 66**).

4. Oligodendroglioma

(a) Accounts for 10% of gliomas, peak age is 35 to 40 years, and there is no sex predominance. The pure form is rare because it is usually mixed with other glial elements (especially astrocytoma).

(b) Symptoms frequently include **seizures**. They grow from the white matter and infiltrate the cortex. CT demonstrates a hypodense lesion that is frequently cystic. It has a higher frequency of **hemorrhage** than other glial tumors (**Fig. 67**).

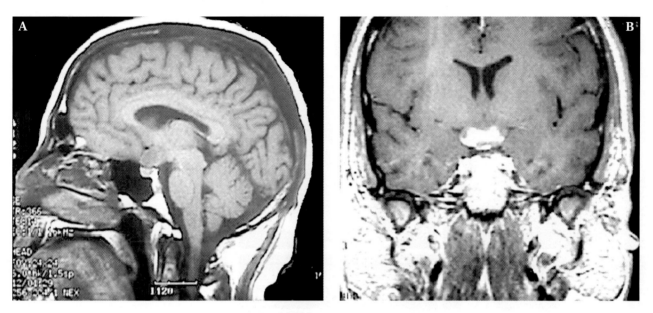

Figure 64   Optic chiasm glioma. T1-weighted noninfused sagittal (A) and infused coronal (B) MRIs demonstrating an expansile enhancing lesion of the optic chiasm.

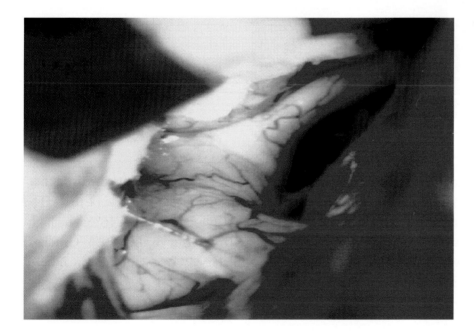

Figure 65   Optic chiasm glioma. Diffuse enlargement with extension under chiasm.

(c) Pathologic examination demonstrates round nuclei with scant cytoplasm, a **chicken-wire vascular pattern** with thin vessels, occasional serpentine configuration, and an Indian-file lineup of cells in the white matter with satelitosis of neurons in the gray matter. The **fried egg yolk**–appearing cells and nucleus are caused by an artifact from cytoplasmic retraction. It is seen in permanent but not in frozen sections. Eighty percent have **calcifications**. Immunohistochemistry is positive for GFAP and S100 (**Fig 68**).

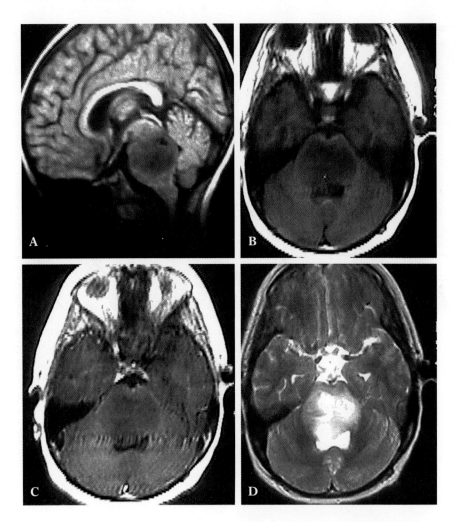

Figure 66   Pontine glioma. T1-weighted sagittal (A), noninfused (B) and infused (C) axial, and T2-weighted axial (D) MRIs with low-intensity nonenhancing expansion of the pons.

(d) Systemic metastases are rare and usually occur after surgery. The 5-year survival is better than for astrocytomas. The most important prognostic factor is grade (1 to 4). The low-grade tumors have a 5-year survival of 74% and 10-year survival of 46%. The high-grade tumors have a 5-year survival of 41% and a 10-year survival of 20%. Grades 3 and 4 have endovascular proliferation and hypercellularity. PCV chemotherapy is helpful for anaplastic oligodendrogliomas.

5. Ependymoma

   (a) Peak age is 10 to 15 years, with a large peak at 1 to 5 years and smaller peak at 35 years. There is no sex predominance.

   (b) Location is usually supratentorial in children and in the **fourth ventricle in adults** (overall in descending order of frequency: fourth ventricle, lateral ventricles, third ventricle, aqueduct, and cerebellopontine angle [CPA]). They may grow from the fourth ventricle and **extrude out through the foramen of Luschka and Magendie**. They also account for **60% of intramedullary spinal cord tumors**, occurring **mostly at the filum**.

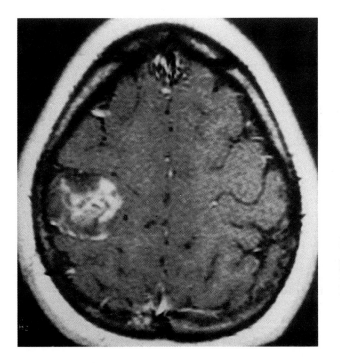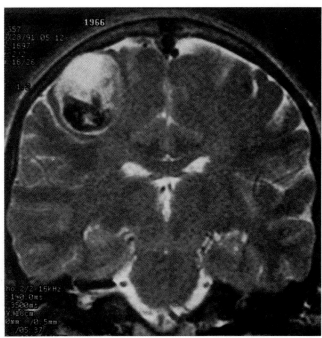

Figure 67   Oligodendroglioma. T1-weighted axial infused (A) and F2-weighted coronal (B) MRIs demonstrating right posterior frontal hemorrhagic tumor.

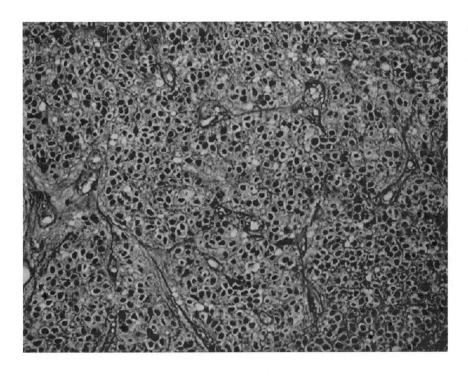

Figure 68   Oligodendroglioma (H and E). Uniform "fried egg" cells with geometric "chicken-wire" arrangement of vessels.

(c) They are usually pencil-shaped in the spinal cord, often associated with a syrinx, and have a good margin for resection. There may be multiple spinal cord tumors with NF2. The **myxopapillary** variety occurs only at the filum (normally it has a good prognosis, but is worse if it invades the conus).

(d) CT and MRI demonstrate a lobulated, circumscribed, cystic, moderately enhancing lesion with calcifications (50%) and only rarely hemorrhage. Grossly it is tan-red in color (**Fig. 69**).

(e) Pathologic examination demonstrates various patterns:

  (i)   Cellular—a sheetlike growth of polygonal cells with **true rosettes** (around a central canal), **pseudorosettes** (around a blood vessel), and **blepharoplasts** (ciliary basal bodies in the apical cytoplasm) (**Fig. 70**).

  (ii) Papillary—with typical papillary projections.

  (iii) Myxopapillary—with intracellular mucin, occurs at the filum and presacral/postsacral area if there is local spread (**Fig. 71**).

  (iv) Clear cell—with oligodendrocyte-like halos.

(f) Immunohistochemistry is positive for GFAP and PTAH. These can be differentiated from: (1) medulloblastoma by the smaller nuclei, less mitoses, absence of Homer Wright rosettes, positive GFAP, and negative synaptophysin and (2) choroid plexus papilloma that are PTAH negative and cytokeratin positive.

(g) Grades 1 and 2 have few mitoses; grade 3 has frequent mitoses and endovascular hyperplasia; and grade 4 has more frequent spinal cord and brain metastases. There is a 45% 5-year survival with prognosis influenced by age, location, and grade. Grades 1 and 2 are better than 3 and 4. Radiation helps prolong survival. A cure is usually only possible with the myxopapillary variant. They frequently seed the CSF, and a subtotal resection is associated with local and distant seeding. Rarely, the presacral and postsacral soft tissue tumors may metastasize to the lung.

(h) Ependymoblastoma occurs in childhood, is in the PNET group, and is malignant.

(i) The normal ependyma consists of a single layer of cuboidal/columnar cells that are ciliated early in life and have microvilli. They have a dual epithelial-glial nature and lie over the subependymal glia.

6. Subependymoma

  (a) Peak age is 40 to 60 years, with male predominance, and it is usually located in the **floor of the inferior fourth ventricle or the septum pellucidum**.

  (b) They arise at the ependymal-subependymal zone and grow slowly. They are benign, avascular, **nonenhancing**, firm, well circumscribed, **hypocellular**, and nodular with **rests of cells** separated by glial fibrils (**Figs. 72 and 73**).

  (c) They contain both **ependymal and astrocytic features** with uniform cells, microcysts, calcifications, vascular hyaline, hemosiderin, and mitoses (without prognostic significance). There is no necrosis, rosettes, or seeding.

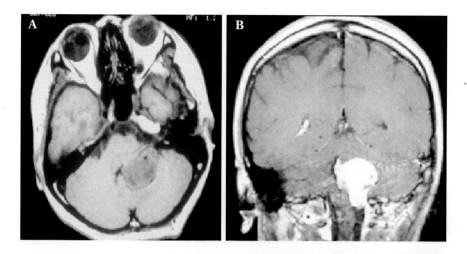

Figure 69   Ependymoma. T1-weighted axial noninfused (A) and coronal infused (B) MRIs demonstrating an enhancing fourth ventricular mass extending through the foramen of Magendie and Luschka.

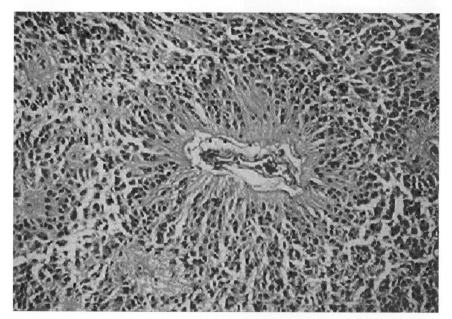

Figure 70   Ependymoma (H and E); pseudorosette (around a vessel).

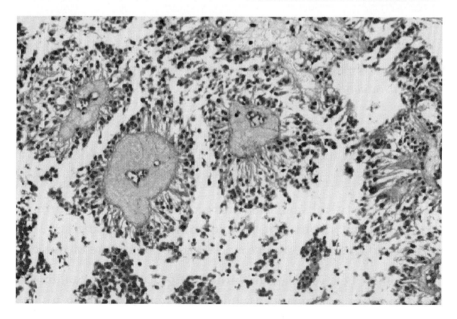

Figure 71   Myxopapillary ependymoma (H and E). Cohesive ependymal cells terminating around mucin-rich perivascular spaces.

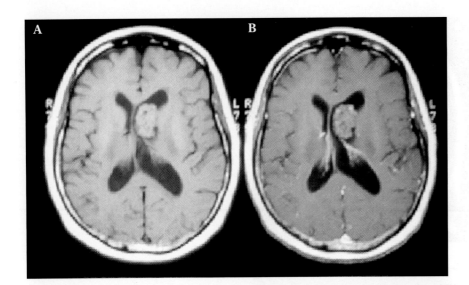

Figure 72   Subependymoma. Noninfused (A) and infused (B) T1-weighted axial MRIs demonstrating a peduculated nonenhancing lateral ventricular mass (the most common location is the fourth ventricle).

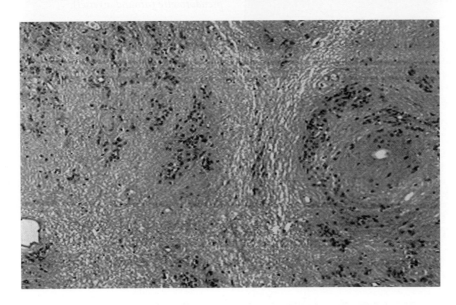

Figure 73   Subependymoma (H and E). Hypocellular with small nests of cells separated by broad bands of fibrils.

      (d) Only 50% become symptomatic, usually by CSF obstruction. A gross total resection can usually be achieved except at the floor of the fourth ventricle. It is postulated that this may be a form of ependymoma because they are often mixed.

  7. Choroid plexus papilloma

      (a) Comprises < 1% of brain tumors and the peak age is < 10 years. It is one of the most frequent tumors before 2 years.

      (b) Fifty percent are located in the lateral ventricle (**more commonly left atrium in children**), 40% are in the **fourth ventricle (more commonly in adults)**, 10% are in the third ventricle, and rarely they are in the CPA. Four percent are bilateral.

      (c) They tend to be well circumscribed, vascular, and **enhancing**. They have a cauliflower papillary shape with cuboidal and columnar cells and no cilia (except in children). The cells are piled up on stalks in a single layer unlike the papillary ependymomas that have multiple layers. Twenty-five percent have calcification. There may be nuclear atypia and rare mitoses, but no mucin. There is rarely bone, cartilage, or melanin formation (**Figs. 74 through 76**).

(d) Immunohistochemisty is positive for transthyretin, vimentin, keratin, S100, and GFAP. It may rarely invade the underlying brain even with benign pathologic findings and may seed the CSF.

(e) Symptoms are usually from **hydrocephalus** as a result of increased CSF production or due to blockage of CSF flow from hemorrhages or direct obstruction. The prognosis does not correlate with the pathologic findings became even benign-appearing tumors may act aggressively.

(f) Surgical resection usually has a good outcome, although there are frequent recurrences. There are rare malignant transformations. Both intraventricular meningiomas and choroid plexus papillomas are more frequently on the left.

(g) The normal choroid is formed from the tela choroidea (the zone of ependymal-pial apposition associated with a fibrovascular stroma) at the floors of the lateral ventricles, the roof of the third ventricle, and the lateral recesses of the fourth ventricle. The tela choroidea is composed of vascular tufts covered by choroid epithelium from the ependyma. The choroid plexus may contain benign cysts or AVMs.

(h) Choroid plexus carcinoma—accounts for 15% of CPPs. They usually occur before 10 years of age, **median age is 2 years**, and they are rare in adults (consider metastasis, especially if EMA is positive, S100 is negative, and vimentin is negative). Most are located in the lateral ventricles and locally invade the parenchyma, as well as seed the CSF. The pathologic findings are less organized, with piled-up epithelium, anaplasia, and necrosis. Treatment is with surgery and radiation with or without chemotherapy. The prognosis is poor (**Fig. 77**).

C. Mixed neuronal and glial tumors (usually a good prognosis)

1. Ganglioglioma—contains both neoplastic neurons and glial cells. 70% occur before 30 years of age. It is usually in the **temporal lobe**, and most commonly presents with **seizures**. It is **well circumscribed, cystic**, firm, and often has a **calcified nodule**. It may enhance. Pathologic examination demonstrates perivascular inflammatory cells, reticulin, **glia**, and **binucleate neurons** with rare mitoses. Immunohistochemistry is positive for neurofilament, **synaptophysin**, neurosecretory granules, and **GFAP** (**Figs. 78 and 79**).

2. Gangliocytoma—neoplastic neurons without neoplastic glia. They may be simply dysplastic brain.

3. Desmoplastic infantile ganglioglioma—rare and usually occur **before 18 months**. They are **massive**, frontal, cystic lesions **adherent to the dura** with a desmoplastic reaction. The tumor enhances. It is differentiated from meningioma because it is GFAP positive and EMA negative.

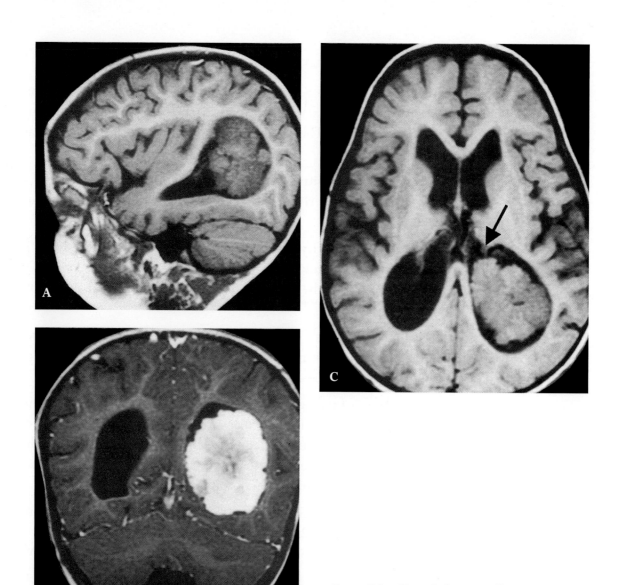

Figure 74   Choroid plexus papilloma. Sagittal (A) and axial (B) non-infused and coronal (C) infused T1-weighted MRIs demonstrating a left lateral ventricular lesion.

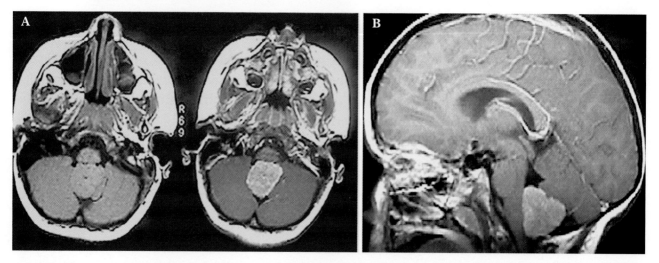

Figure 75   Choroid plexus papilloma. Axial noninfused (A) and infused (B) and sagittal infused T1-weighted MRIs demonstrating a fourth ventricular enhancing mass (more common in the left lateral ventricle in children and the fourth ventricle in adults).

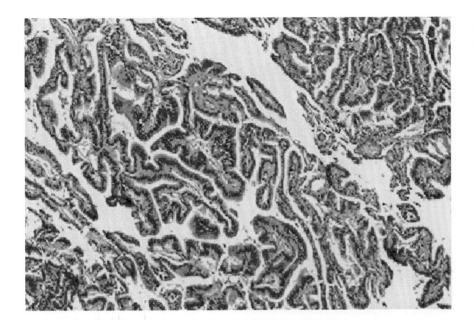

Figure 76   Choroid plexus papilloma (H and E). Fairly well-ordered columnar cells resting on a delicate fibrovascular stroma.

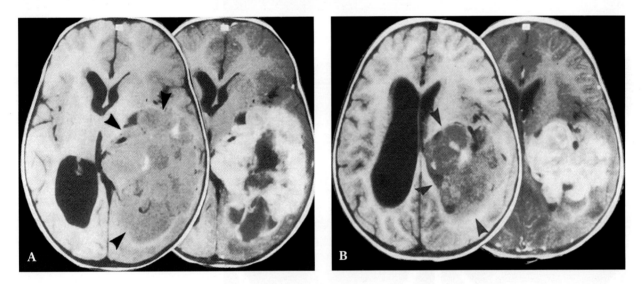

Figure 77   Choroid plexus carcinoma. Axial non-infused and infused T1-weighted MRIs (A and B) demonstrating a large enhancing left intraventricular lesion with parenchymal extension.

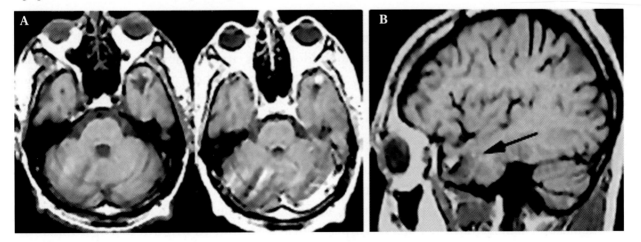

Figure 78   Ganglioglioma. Axial noninfused (A) and infused (B) and sagittal infused T1-weighted MRIs demonstrating a cystic lesion in the left temporal tip with an enhancing mural nodule.

67

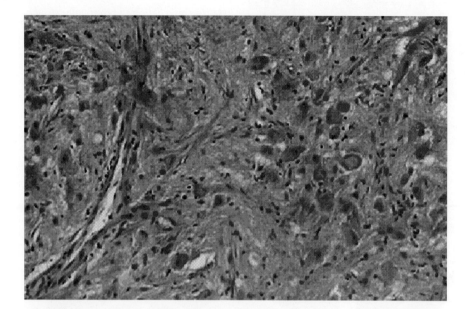

Figure 79   Ganglioglioma (H and E). Clusters of abnormal-appearing neurons (some are binucleated) in a backround of neoplastic glial tissue.

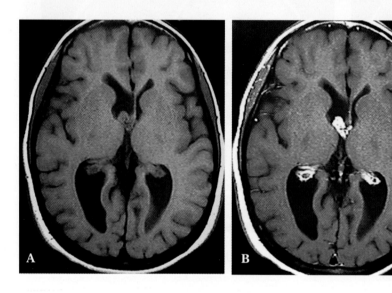

Figure 80   Central neurocytoma. Axial T1-weighted noninfused (A) and infused (B) MRIs demonstrate enhancing mass near the septum pellucidum and foramen of Monro.

4. Dysembryoplastic neuroepithelial tumor—usually in people 1 to 19 years of age, presents with seizures, and is located in the temporal lobe. It is circumscribed, cystic, multinodular, superficial, and cortical. It contains normal neurons with abnormal oligodendrocytes and astrocytes (a ganglioglioma has abnormal neurons, is in the white matter, and lacks nodularity). It is associated with cortical dysplasia. Surgical resection is usually curative and radiation is not needed.

5. Central neurocytoma—occurs in young adults, usually originates at the **septum pellucidum** and occurs in the lateral and third ventricles near the foramen of Monroe. It is circumscribed, **lobulated**, **enhancing**, noninfiltrative, and usually contains **calcifications**. Pathologic examination demonstrates monotonous hypercellularity **similar to oligodendrogliomas** with rare mitoses, frequent cysts and necrosis, and occasionally hemorrhage. Immunohistochemistry is positive for **synaptophysin** (**Figs. 80 and 81**).

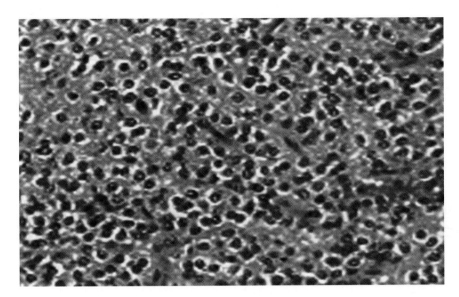

Figure 81   Central neurocytoma (H and E). Closely packed uniform undifferentiated cells with small blue nuclei and perinuclear halos. The histologic findings are similar to oligodendroglioma, but central neurocytoma stains with synaptophysin and neuron-specific enolase.

D. Primitive neuroectodermal tumors (PNETs)

1. *Medulloblast*—a term originally coined by Bailey and Cushing in 1925 to describe **bipotential cells** capable of differentiating into glia or neurons. These cells have features similar to the totipotent neural tube cells. It is postulated that they are derived from the external granular layer of the cerebellum or from dysplastic cell rests in the anterior and posterior medullary velum. The term *PNET* was introduced by Hart and Earle in 1973.

2. PNET varieties

   (a) Medulloblastoma—50% occur before 10 years and 75% before 15 years, and there is a second peak at 28 years. There is a male predominance and they are more frequently off the midline in adults. They account for 20% of CNS tumors in children and one-third of the posterior fossa tumors in children. They are associated with basal cell nevus syndrome.

   (b) Retinoblastoma—the most common extracranial malignant solid tumor in children and 80% occur before 5 years. It is derived from a neural crest precursor of the sympathetic ganglia. There is a genetic predisposition by loss of a suppressor gene. It is treated with surgery and radiation. Retinoblastomas contain **Flexner-Wintersteiner** and Homer Wright rosettes. **Trilateral retinoblastoma is bilateral retinoblastoma with pineoblastoma.**

   (c) Pineoblastoma (see Section I on Pineal Tumors)

   (d) Ependymoblastoma

   (e) Spongioblastoma (glial)

   (f) Central neuroblastoma—usually supratentorial, hemispheric, and circumscribed. It usually occurs before 5 years. It may be hemorrhagic, necrotic, and cystic. The survival is 30% in 5 years. Neuroblastoma is the third most common tumor in children after leukemia and brain tumor. Two percent involve the brain. It is frequently congenital and make up 18% of tumors in patients < 2 months old. Peripheral neuroblastoma develops in the adrenal gland in children and may have spinal epidural metastases.

(g) Medulloepithelioma—derived from ventricular matrix cells, is the most primitive of the PNETs, and affects very young children.

3. PNET features

(a) Locations (in descending order of frequency)—**vermis**, cerebellar hemispheres (older children), pineal, cerebrum, spinal cord, and brain stem.

(b) PNETs are **hyperdense on CT**, hypointense on T1-weighted MRI, and enhancing (**Fig. 82**).

(c) They are pink-brown in color and may be soft or firm. They occasionally hemorrhage, are rarely calcified, and are frequently cystic (80%). They have no capsule, are occasionally circumscribed, and **frequently disseminate in the CSF**. PNETs are **densely cellular**, contain **small round cells with large nuclei and scant cytoplasm**, have a variable number of mitoses, and occasional necrosis (**Fig. 83**). There are **Homer Wright rosettes** (around central granulofibrillar material with radially arranged nuclei), pseudorosettes (around blood vessels), ependymal canals (especially with ependymoblastoma), and **Flexner–Wintersteiner rosettes** (columnar cells with a small lumen seen with retinoblastomas and also pinealblastomas) (**Figs. 84 through 86**). There may be a linear array of cells Indian file and **round islands of cells**. There are occasional astrocytes and oligodendrocytes. Neurons can be stained with silver, PTAH, etc. There rarely may be smooth or striated muscle cells or melanocytes.

(d) **Fifty percent of these tumors metastasize** (two-third sin the CNS and one-third **to bone**), and 20 to 50% are disseminated at the time of diagnosis. The survival is > 50% at 5 years with surgery, chemotherapy, and radiation therapy. Complete resection provides 75% 5-year and 25% 10-year survivals.

E. Meningiomas—account for 15% of primary intracranial tumors. Peak age is 40 to 60 years. **Females** are more commonly affected. **Seventy-two percent of tumors have monosomy 22.**

1. Meningioma incidence is increased by **radiation** and the presence of neurofibromatosis type 2 (**NF2**). Younger patients more likely have the malignant papillary variant or hemangiopericytoma.

2. Meningiomas have hormone receptors for **estrogen**, progesterone, peptides, amines, androgen, glucocortisone, somatostatin, and CCK. They may grow with pregnancy and breast cancer.

3. The blood supply is from **external carotid artery (ECA)** branches such as the middle meningeal and anterior falcine arteries. They may parasitize pial vessels (from the ICA) and develop a dual supply. They invade dura and bone. Bony changes are hyperostotic more frequently than lytic. The hyperostotic bone usually has evidence of invasion by tumor.

4. Meningiomas rarely metastasize. They originate from the **arachnoid cap cells** (these also form whorls and psammoma bodies) that are most frequently located at the arachnoid

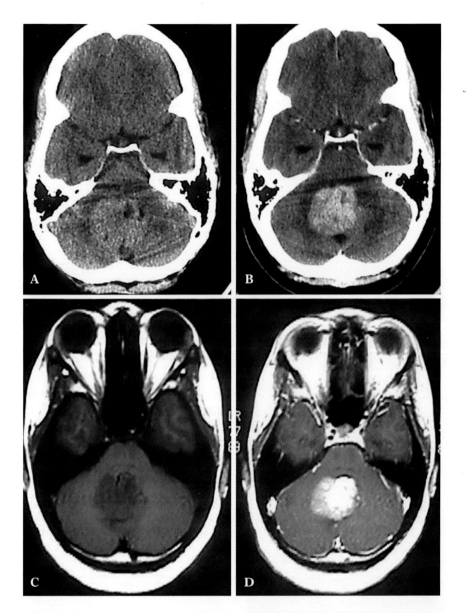

Figure 82   Medulloblastoma. Axial CT noninfused (A) and infused (B) and axial T1-weighted MRI noninfused (C) and infused (D) demonstrating a slightly hyperdense and hypointense enhancing mass.

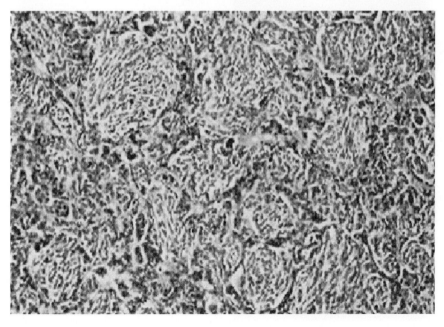

Figure 83   Medulloblastoma (H and E). Closely packed undifferentiated cells with no discernible cytoplasm (small blue cells) with islands of more loosely packed cells.

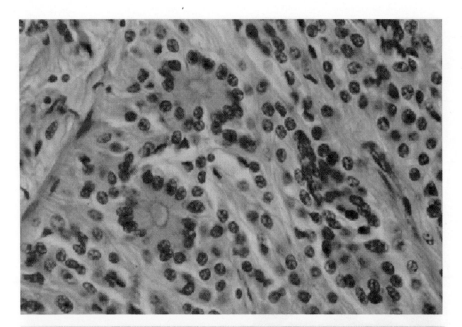

Figure 84   True "ependymal" rosette (H and E). Polar ependymal cells with basal bodies of cilia (blepharoplasts) lining a central lumen; most commonly in ependymoma. (See Figure 28.)

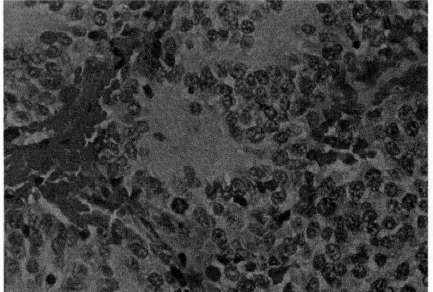

Figure 85   Homer Wright rosette (H and E). Central fibrillar material (processes of tumor cells) ringed by radially arranged cell nuclei; most commonly seen with medulloblastoma and neuroblastoma.

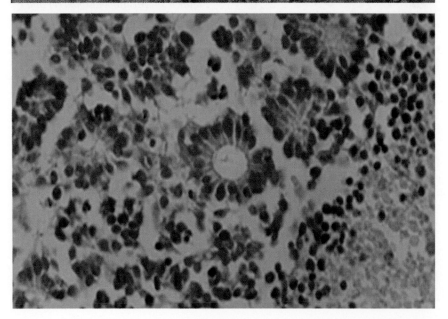

Figure 86   Flexner-Wintersteiner rosette (H and E). Columnar cells that resemble cone-type photoreceptor cells form rosettes with small central lumens; most commonly in pineal tumors and also retinoblastoma.

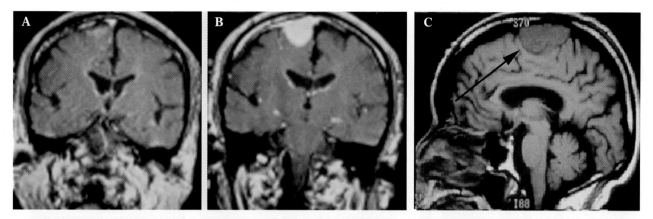

Figure 87   Parasagittal meningioma. Noninfused (A) and infused (B) coronal and **noninfused sagittal (C)** *T1-weighted MRIs demonstrating a homogenously enhancing circumscribed isotense lesion arising from the medial dura and invading the wall of the superior sagittal sinus.*

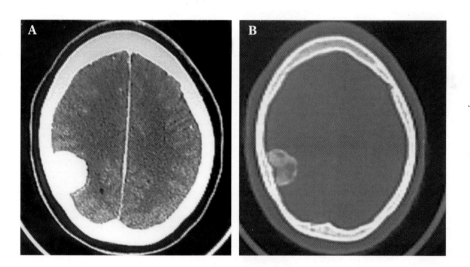

Figure 88   Convexity meningioma. Axial infused (A) and bone window (B) CTs demonstrating a homogenously enhancing, circumscribed, calcified lesion arising from the convexity.

granulations (near the superior sagittal sinus under the suture confluence) and the tela choroidea (intraventricular).

5. Locations—cranial (90%), spinal (9%), and ectopic (1%, intraosseous skull, orbit, neck, scalp, sinus, and parotid). Cranial locations in descending order are **parasagittal** (middle $\frac{1}{3}$ of the superior sagittal sinus), convexity (near the coronal suture), sphenoid tuberculum, olfactory groove, foramen magnum, optic nerve, tentorial, choroid (left lateral ventricle), and thoracic. The parasagittal and convexity group accounts for 50% (**Figs. 87 through 92**) .

6. They are **multiple** in 9% of cases. Metastatic cancer has been reported inside of a meningioma.

7. Pathologically, they are well demarcated and usually firm and rubbery. The shape may be globular or en plaque. Radiographically, 10% are cystic, 25% have calcifications, 90% enhance, 75% are hyperdense on CT and 25% are isodense on CT.

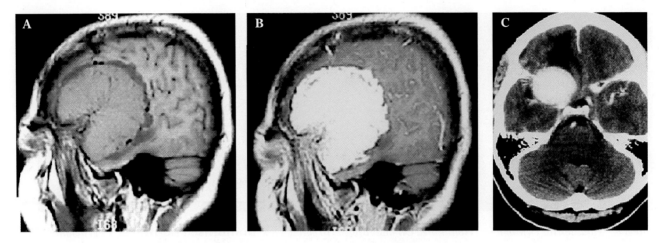

Figure 89   Sphenoid wing meningioma. Sagittal noninfused (A) and infused (B) T1-weighted MRIs and (C) axial infused CT demonstrating a homogenously enhancing circumscribed lesion arising from the sphenoid ridge.

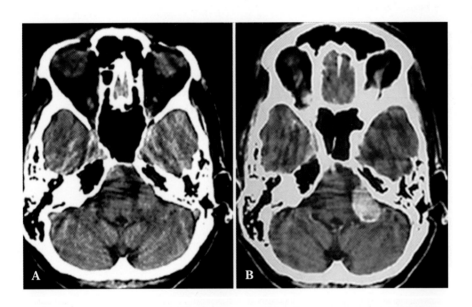

Figure 90   CPA meningioma. Axial noninfused (A) and infused (B) CTs demonstrating the dural-based enhancing left-sided mass.

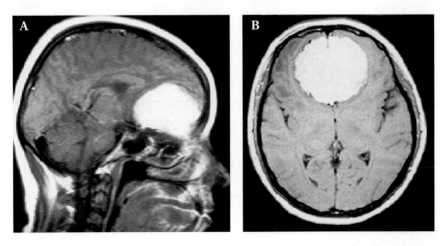

Figure 91   Olfactory groove meningioma. Infused sagittal (A) and axial (B) T1-weighted MRIs demonstrating a homogenously enhancing circumscribed lesion arising from the floor of the anterior fossa.

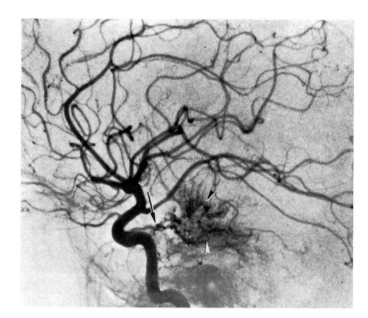

*Figure 92   Tentorial meningioma. Angiogram demonstrates the tumor blush of the meningioma with supply by an enlarged **tentorial artery of Bernasconi-Cassinari**.*

8. There is a sunburst pattern of dural feeders, basophillic **psammoma bodies**, and **whorls (Figs. 93 and 94)**. Immunohistochemistry is of mesenchymal and epithelial cells, positive for both **vimentin and EMA**.

9. Variants include: (1) meningothelial or syncytial with whorls, lobules, but few psammoma bodies; (2) fibroblastic with sheets of cells; (3) transitional (the most common type) containing elements of both the syncytial and fibroblastic types; (4) psammomatous; and (5) angiomatous. These variants do not affect the prognosis, and nuclear atypia is common. Ninety-two percent of meningiomas are "typical." The atypical group (6%) has at least two of the following: hypercellularity, frequent mitoses, and necrosis. There is no brain invasion. They have a 30% 5-year survival, 50% recur in 1.5 years, and 5% metastasize.

10. The anaplastic or malignant group (2%) either invades the brain, metastasizes, is papillary (especially in younger patients), has necrosis, or increased mitoses. Seventy percent of these recur and 30% metastasize.

11. **Foster-Kennedy syndrome**—optic atrophy in one eye and papilledema in the other with anosmia, seen occasionally with olfactory groove meningiomas (**Figs. 95 and 96**).

F. Hemangiopericytoma—it represents 2.5% of diagnosed meningiomas. It used to be considered a type of meningioma but now is believed to be a distinct entity. Mean age is 40 to 50 years with a **male predominance**.

1. They are usually supratentorial.

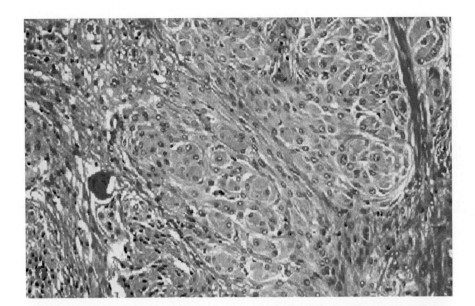

Figure 93   Meningioma (H and E); synctial pattern and a psammoma body.

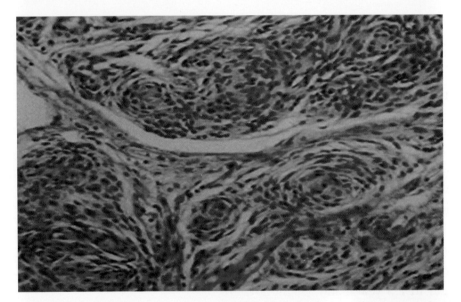

Figure 94   Meningioma (H and E); whorls.

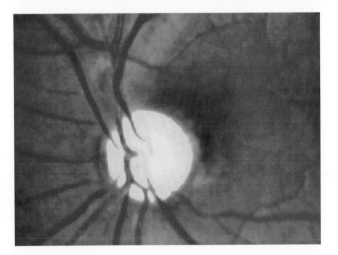

Figure 95   Optic atrophy; severe optic disc pallor.

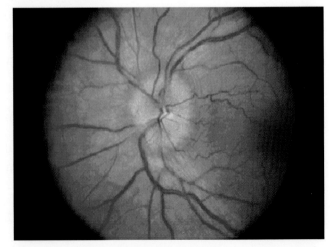

Figure 96   Papilledema; obscured optic disc margins.

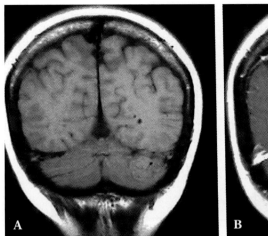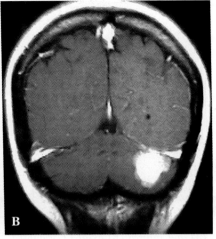

Figure 97   Hemangiopericytoma. T1-weighted coronal noninfused (A) and infused (B) MRIs demonstrating an enhancing circumscribed mass inferior to the tentorium.

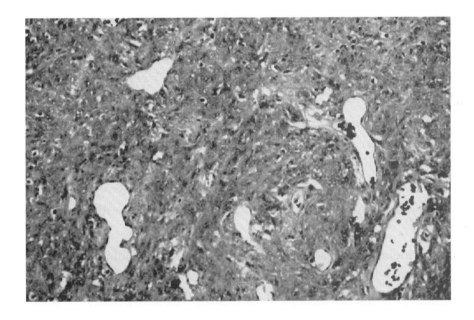

Figure 98   Hemangiopericytoma (H and E). Densely cellular with "staghorn" vascular spaces.

2. The 5-, 10-, and 15-year survivals are 63%, 37%, and 21%, respectively. Recurrence rate is 70%. Ten to 30% metastasize, especially to lung and bone. They respond poorly to radiation and chemotherapy.

3. They are postulated to originate from pericyte cells that contract and surround capillaries. They are dural based, well demarcated, firm, and vascular (**Fig. 97**).

4. The blood supply is usually from the **ICA** or vertebrobasilar systems.

5. Pathologic findings are dense cellularity with frequent mitoses, increased reticulin, lobules around **"staghorn" vascular channels**, and **absence of whorls or psammoma bodies**. Immunohistochemistry is positive for vimentin but **not EMA** (positive in meningiomas) (**Fig. 98**).

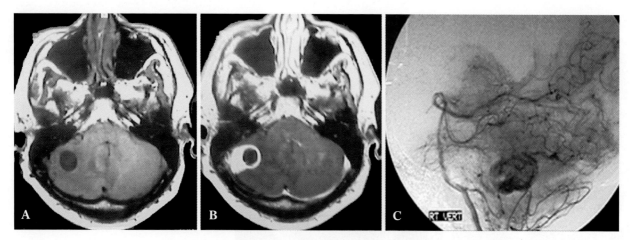

Figure 99   Hemangioblastoma. Noninfused (A) and infused (B) axial T1-weighted MRIs demonstrating a cystic lesion with enhancement of rim and mural nodule and (C) lateral basilar artery angiogram with filling of a different hemangioblastoma.

G. Hemangioblastoma—it accounts for 2% of intracranial tumors and 10% of posterior fossa tumors. Mean age is 20 to 40 years with a **male predominance**.

  1. The most common locations are cerebellar hemispheres or vermis (80%), cervical spinal cord (10%), and brain stem (3%).

  2. Sixty percent are **cystic with an enhancing mural nodule abutting the pia** and 40% are solid (**Fig. 99**). In the spinal cord, they are frequently associated with a syrinx. They tend to be circular, yellow (secondary to lipid content), and contain capillaries with hyperplastic endothelial cells and pericytes surrounded by **stromal cells with vacuoles** and lipids (**Fig. 100**).

  3. Hemangioblastomas are rich in **reticulin,** have no mitoses, and rarely have calcifications, hemorrhage, or necrosis.

  4. They can be differentiated from metastatic renal cell carcinoma because immunohistochemistry is positive for vimentin and negative for EMA.

  5. There is occasional polycythemia caused the tumor's **erythropoietin secretion**.

  6. Surgery is usually curative, although the recurrence rate is 25%. Eighty percent are sporadic and 20% are associated with Von Hippel Lindau Syndrome (**VHL**).

H. Craniopharyngioma—it accounts for 2 to 5% of primary tumors. There is no sex predominance. Peak age is 0 to 20 years with a second peak at 50 years. Seventy percent are suprasellar and intrasellar and they are rarely exclusively sellar, CPA, pineal, or nasopharyngeal.

  1. The tumor is benign, but it invades into vital structures. It is derived from squamous cells from **Rathke's cleft**. It is usually a cyst with a nodule filled with **"machine oil" fluid** and cholesterol crystals that can elicit a granulomatous reaction.

  2. It contains **calcifications** in 90% (100% in children and 50% in adults), usually enhances, and has sharp irregular margins with surrounding gliosis (**Fig. 101**).

  3. Pathologic examination demonstrates an **adamantinomatous** pattern with rests of epithelial cells surrounded by a layer of columnar basal cells separated by a myxoid stroma of

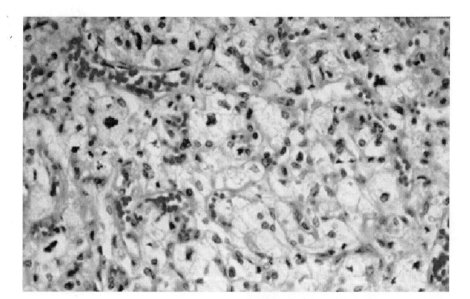

Figure 100   Hemangioblastoma (H and E). Abundant thin-walled vascular channels interspersed with enlarged vacuolated stromal cells.

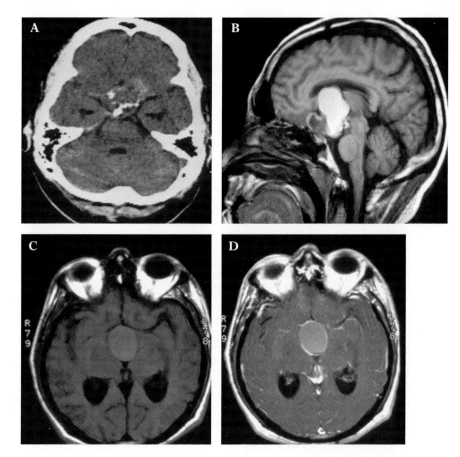

Figure 101   Craniopharyngioma. Non-infused axial CT (A) demonstrating calcifications, sagittal T1-weighted MRI (B) with hyperintense cyst, and T1-weighted MRIs noninfused (C) and infused (D) with rim enhancement.

loose stellate cells, whorls of cells, and keratinized nodules of wet keratin (**Figs. 101 through 104**).

4. They may contain teeth, as found in jaw tumors. There is a papillary variant that is usually in adults, located in the third ventricle, solid, without calcifications, and contains papillae of well-differentiated squamous epithelium. This tumor has a better prognosis.

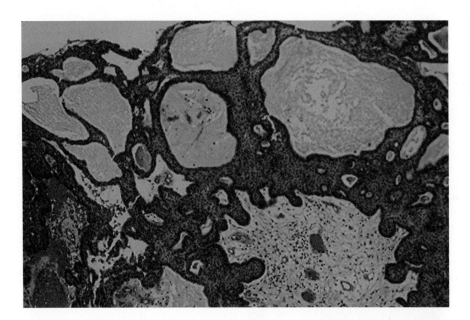

Figure 102   Craniopharyngioma (H and E). "Adamantinomatous" pattern with basaloid layer of cells separated by loosely arranged stellate cells.

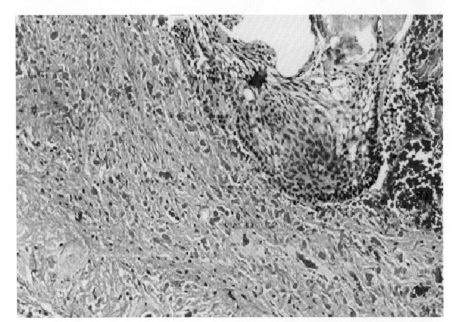

Figure 103   Craniopharyngioma (H and E). "Adamantinomatous" pattern with basaloid layer of cells separated by loosely arranged stellate cells. Higher power view.

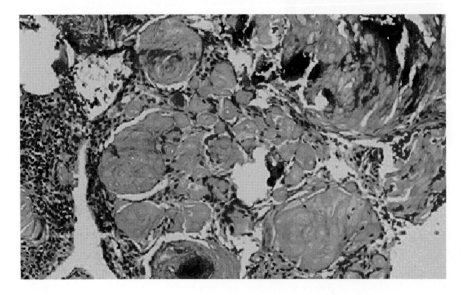

Figure 104   Craniopharyngioma (H and E). Billowed "wet" keratin and calcifications.

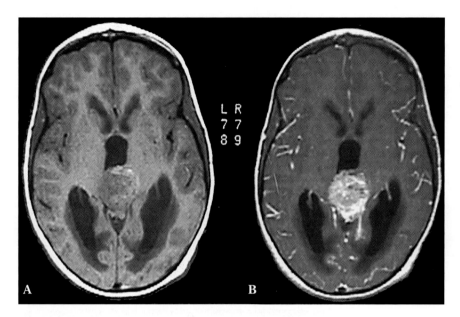

Figure 105   Pineocytoma. Axial non-infused (A) and infused (B) T1-weighted MRIs demonstrating enhancing, demarcated, posterior third ventricular mass.

I. Pineal tumors

1. General information

(a) The pineal gland contains pinealocytes (derived from APUD cells) and astrocytes. It is usually calcified by age 16 years. In reptiles, it functions as a photoreceptor to change skin color in response to light. In humans, it is involved with hormone secretion for circadian rhythms.

(b) It is innervated by **sympathetic nerves** from the superior cervical ganglion that release **NE** to increase the pineal gland's **melatonin** secretion. The pineal gland inhibits gonadal development and regulates menstruation, adrenal function, and thyroid function.

(c) Pineal tumors account for 1% of intracranial tumors in the United States and 6% in Japan. Pineal tumors may be derived from pineal cells (20%; includes pineocytoma and pineoblastoma), interstitial cells (rare; usually well differentiated astrocytes), and germ cells (the most frequent pineal tumor).

(d) **Trilateral retinoblastoma** is bilateral retinoblastomas with a pinealblastoma. Pineal masses may compress the tectum and cause **Parinaud's syndrome** with poor upgaze, pupillary dilation, lid retraction, nystagmus retractorius, and dissociated near-light response (reaction to near but not light).

2. Pineocytoma—peak age is 30 years and there is no sex predominance. It is well circumscribed, contained within the gland, with medium-sized round cells, and **Homer Wright rosettes** with central fibrillar material. There is a better outcome if there is some neuronal and/or astrocytic differentiation. There is rarely metastasis and CSF dissemination (**Figs. 105 and 106**).

3. Pineoblastoma—a member of the PNET group with peak age < 20 years. It infiltrates surrounding structures, **disseminates in the CSF**, and metastasizes to bone, lung, and lymph

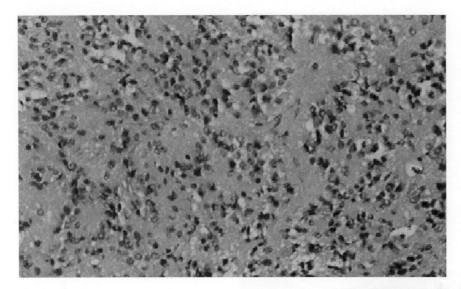

Figure 106   Pineocytoma (H and E). Rosettelike clusters of nuclei surrounding fibrillary neuropil-like matrix recapitulating normal pineal parenchyma.

nodes. It enhances well. It is hypercellular and has small cells, mitoses, and necrosis. The mean survival is < 2 years (**Figs. 107 and 108**).

J.   Germ cell tumors (**Table 1**)

1. General information

    (a) Mean age is 10 to 20 years (at the onset of puberty in males).

    (b) These cells originate in the yolk sac endoderm and migrate throughout the embryo.

    (c) The most frequent locations include pineal, suprasellar (especially in females), third ventricular, posterior fossa, and the midline mediastinum and retroperitoneum.

2. Germinoma—the **most common pineal tumor** (40%) and accounts for two-thirds of germ cell tumors. Peak age is 10 to 30 years and there is a **male predominance**.

    (a) It is usually in the pineal region, although the **second most common site is suprasellar and intrasellar**. Ten percent are both in the pineal and suprasellar regions.

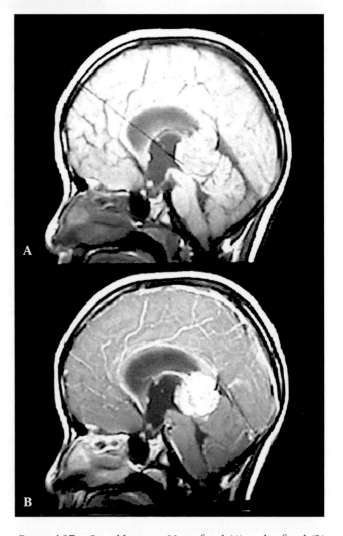

Figure 107   Pineoblastoma. Noninfused (A) and infused (B) sagittal T1-weighted MRIs demonstrating a fairly circumscribed, enhancing pineal region mass.

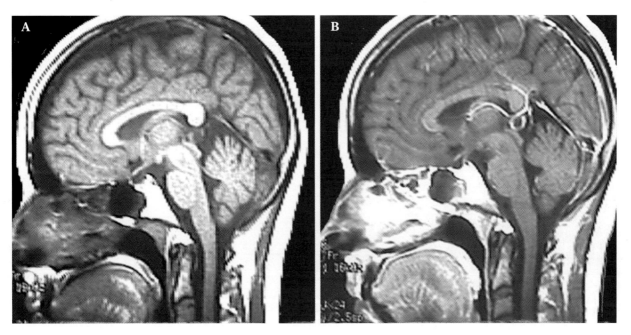

Figure 108   Pineal cyst. Sagittal T1-weighted noninfused (A) and infused (B) MRIs demonstrating a cystic expansion of the pineal gland.

TABLE 1. GERM CELL TUMOR DERIVATION

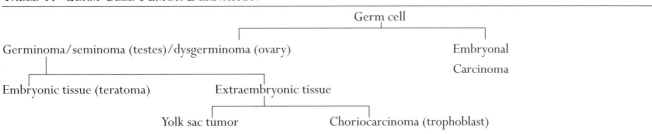

		Germ cell		
Germinoma/seminoma (testes)/dysgerminoma (ovary)				Embryonal Carcinoma
Embryonic tissue (teratoma)		Extraembryonic tissue		
	Yolk sac tumor		Choriocarcinoma (trophoblast)	

(b) It is soft with **large polygonal cells** and lacks necrosis or hemorrhage. There is an **infiltrate of T cells with follicles (Fig. 109)**.

(c) It is isointense on T1-weighted MRI, hypointense on T2-weighted MRI, and hyperdense on CT. It enhances well (**Fig. 110**).

(d) There is an occasional increase in serum βHCG, but this may be due to an associated component of choriocarcinoma. In males, it is associated with precocious puberty.

(e) Treatment is with **radiation** to the entire neuroaxis.

3. Embryonal carcinoma—rare, contains necrosis and hemorrhage, and has elevated serum **AFP** and βHCG.

4. Yolk sac tumor (endodermal sinus tumor)—rare, occurs in young children, and has elevated serum **AFP** and Schiller-Duval bodies.

5. Choriocarcinoma—may be primary or metastatic. Primary usually occurs in the first decade of life. It has a high propensity to **hemorrhage** because of thin-walled vessels. Serum is positive for **βHCG**. Prognosis is poor.

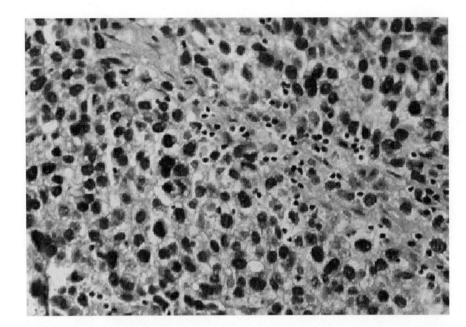

Figure 109   Germinoma (H and E). Large polygonal cells with large nuclei and prominent nucleoli and T-cell infiltrates.

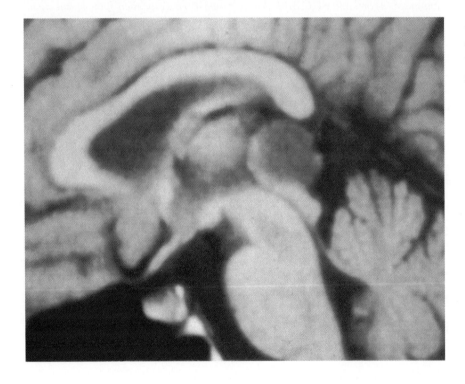

Figure 110   Pineal region germinoma. Sagittal noninfused T1-weighted MRI with low-intensity demarcated pineal mass.

5. Teratoma—the second most common pineal germ cell tumor (15%). It usually affects **young males**. It contains tissues from all three layers: skin, nerve, cartilage, bone, fat, muscle, respiratory glands, and GI glands. There may be elevated serum **CEA** (**Fig. 111**).

6. Alfa-fetoprotein (AFP)—secreted by mucous glands of the GI tract and elevated with yolk sac tumors and hepatic carcinomas.

7. βHCG—synthesized by the placenta and elevated with choriocarcinoma.

K. Pituitary tumors

1. They account for 15% of intracranial tumors. Mean age is 20 to 50 years. There is a **female predominance** with PR- and ACTH-secreting tumors and a **male predominance** with GH-secreting tumors. Twenty-five percent of these tumors do not secrete hormone.

2. **Microadenomas** are < 1 cm and are much more common than **macroadenomas**. Pituitary tumors are associated with **MEN type I**. Less than 1% are malignant, and metastases are more frequent than primary malignancies in the sella.

3. H & E staining reveals acidophils (40%; PR, GH, and FSH/LH), **basophils (10%; ACTH, and TSH)**, and null cells (50%) (**Fig. 112**).

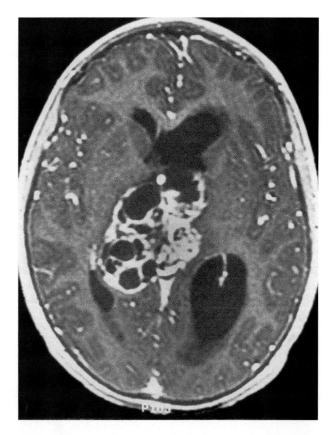

Figure 111   Pineal teratoma. Axial T1-weighted infused MRI demonstrating lobulated cystic pineal mass with irregular enhancement.

4. CT and T1-weighted MRI are isodense/isointense with **decreased enhancement** of the tumor compared with the normal pituitary gland. The T2-weighted MRI may be hypointense. Angiogram may demonstrate an enlarged meningohypophyseal trunk, and 4 to 7% of pituitary tumors are associated with intracranial aneurysms (**Figs. 113 and 114**).

5. Forty percent have local invasion at the time of diagnosis. Recurrence after surgery is 16% at 8 years and 35% at 20 years.

6. PR-secreting tumor is the **most common pituitary tumor** (30%). Symptoms include **amenorrhea/galactorrhea** in women and decreased libido or impotence in men. The tumors tend to be larger and patients older in men. The serum PR level is > 150 and is proportional to tumor size. These tumors respond well to **bromocriptine** (a dopamine agonist). The prolactin may be elevated because of decreased dopamine (prolactin inhibitory factor; PIF) from compression on the pituitary stalk from a nonprolactinoma (**"stalk effect"**).

7. GH-secreting tumor is the second most common pituitary hormone—secreting tumor (13%). It causes **acromegaly** in adults and gigantism in children. Forty percent also have increased

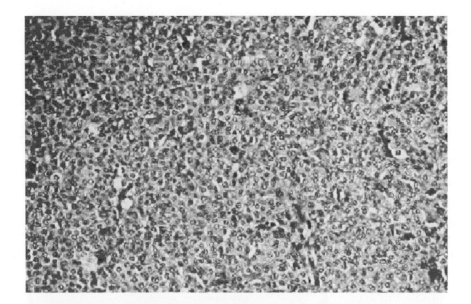

Figure 112   Pituitary adenoma (H and E). Diffuse pattern of monotonous polygonal cells.

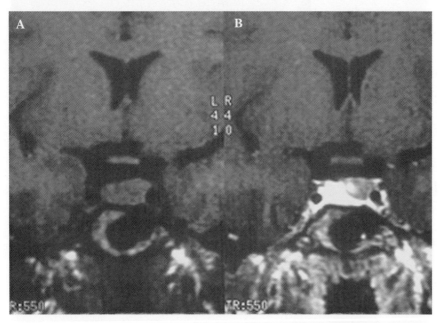

Figure 113   Pituitary microadenoma. Noninfused (A) and infused (B) coronal T1-weighted MRIs demonstrating the left-sided nonenhancing lesion.

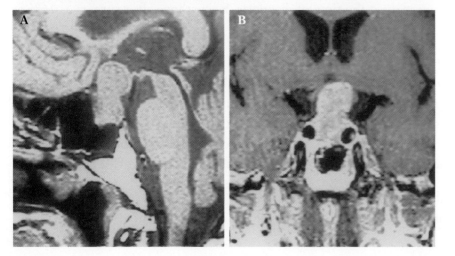

Figure 114   Pituitary macroadenoma. Noninfused sagittal (A) and infused coronal (B) T1-weighted MRIs demonstrating an enhancing lesion filling the sella and suprasellar space, displacing the optic tracts, and invading into the cavernous sinus.

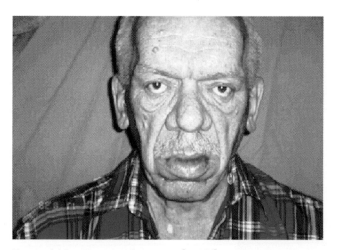

Figure 115   *Acromegaly; coarse facial features.*

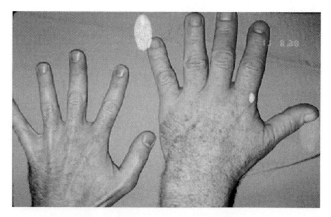

Figure 116   *Acromegaly; enlargement of hand.*

serum PR and TSH. Treatment is surgical or with octreotide (somatostatin analog) (**Figs. 115 and 116**).

8. ACTH-secreting tumor accounts for 10% of pituitary tumors. It is more common in females and produces **Cushing's disease**. **Nelson's syndrome** occurs when there is pituitary enlargement after adrenalectomy (that was performed mistakenly for hypercortisolism thought to be peripherally mediated or as treatment for known Cushing's disease). This tumor is characterized by **Crooke's hyaline change** in the pituitary gland by the accumulation of intermediate filaments in the nontumoral corticotrophs in the presence of elevated steroid levels. Treatment is surgical.

9. FSH/LH-secreting tumor accounts for 9% of pituitary tumors and has no sex predominance. It occurs mostly in the elderly and causes compressive symptoms, although occasionally infertility in women.

10. TSH-secreting tumor accounts for 1% of pituitary tumors.

11. Null cell tumor (oncocytoma) accounts for 26% of pituitary tumors and is the second most common after PR.

12. Pituitary apoplexy—hemorrhagic necrosis of a pituitary adenoma when it outgrows its blood supply. It usually occurs with null cell macroadenomas. It is detected in 1% of pituitary adenomas while patients are alive, but in 10% of tumors at autopsy. Treatment is with surgery and steroid replacement.

13. Lymphocytic hypophysitis—pituitary insufficiency in **peripartum females** caused by an autoimmune mechanism with humoral and cellular components (B and T cells involved). There may also be inflammation in the ovaries and thyroid. Treatment is by surgical decompression if necessary and hormone replacement (**Figs. 117 and 118**).

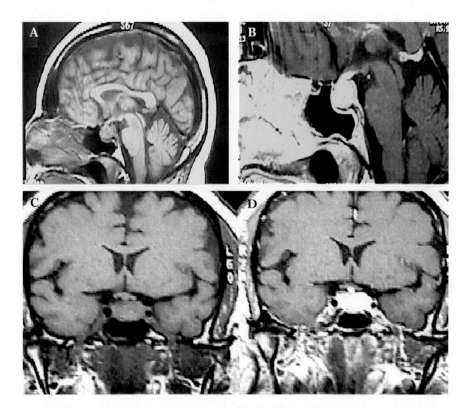

Figure 117   Lymphocytic hypophysitis. Sagittal noninfused (A) and infused (B) and coronal noninfused (C) and infused (D) T1-weighted MRIs demonstrating irregular enhancement and diffuse enlargement of the pituitary gland and infundibulum.

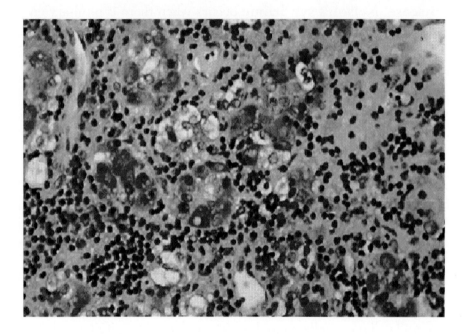

Figure 118   Lymphocytic hypophysitis (H and E). Lymphocytes infiltrating into the pituitary gland.

14. Giant cell pituitary granuloma—characterized by noncaseating, granulomas, no sex predominance. It occurs in adults and is not associated with pregnancy.

15. Empty sella syndrome—**primary** is from the incomplete development of the diaphragma sella. The arachnoid bulges into the sella and may compress the pituitary gland. There may be

an enlarged sella. **Secondary** occurs after radiation, surgery, stroke, or intrapartum shock with ischemic necrosis of the anterior pituitary gland (**Sheehan's syndrome**).

16. Rathke's cleft cyst—it usually occurs in women ages 30 to 40 years. It is a **remnant of the craniopharyngeal duct** that develops when the proximal part closes early and the distal cleft remains open between the pars distalis and pars nervosa. **Seventy percent are both suprasellar and intrasellar.** It is usually >1 cm. Symptoms include visual changes and increased PR. The CT is hypodense and the **T1-weighted MRI is hyporintense**. Fifty percent have rim

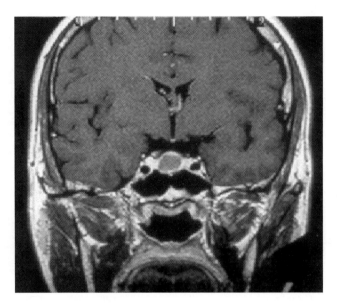

Figure 119   Rathke's cleft cyst. Infused T1-weighted coronal MRI demonstrating a low-intensity cystic lesion in the sella.

enhancement. There are **no calcifications**. It contains watery mucous fluid lined with goblet ciliated cells and columnar/cuboidal epithelial cells (**Fig. 119**).

L. Epidermoid tumor

1. It accounts for 1% of primary tumors. Peak age is 30 to 50 years and there is no sex predominance.

2. Intracranial locations in descending order of frequency include **CPA** (50%), suprasellar, intraventricular, and thalamic. Ten percent are extradural-intradiploic. It is the **third most common CPA lesion** after vestibular schwannomas and meningiomas.

3. On CT and MRI, the tumor's density/intensity is **similar to CSF** and there is no enhancement (**Fig. 120**).

4. It is smooth, encapsulated, has a **pearly sheen**, and contains dry, flaky keratin and stratified cuboidal squamous epithelium (**Figs. 121 and 122**). The progressive desquamation of the cyst wall causes a **linear growth rate**. Fifteen percent have calcifications. It rarely ruptures and frequently recurs after surgery.

5. An epidermoid tumor insinuates along the basal cisterns. An arachnoid cyst can be ruled out by diffusion-weighted MRI that shows the epidermoid to be more like parenchyma than CSF.

6. It develops from ectoderm elements that become trapped intracranially. Epidermoids may form in the lumbosacral spine after lumbar puncture, especially if the stylet of the needle is not in place allowing skin elements to be deposited into deep layers.

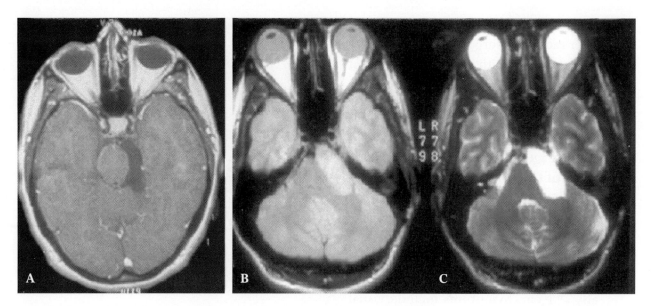

Figure 120   Epidermoid tumor. Infused T1-weighted (A), proton density (B), and T2-weighted (C) axial MRIs demonstrating a low-density lesion in the cisterns along the left side of the brain stem.

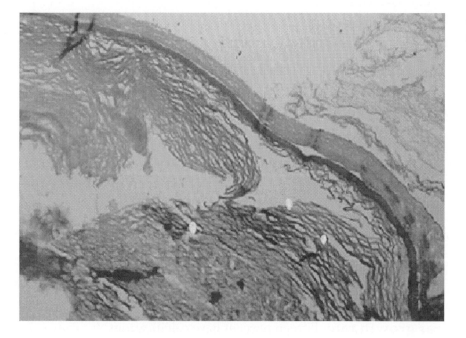

Figure 121   Epidermoid cyst (H and E); thin "dry" keratin.

7. **Mollaret's meningitis** is a recurring **aseptic meningitis** with large cells in the CSF. It occurs in some patients with epidermoid tumors.

M. Dermoid tumor

1. It accounts for 0.1% of primary tumors. There is no sex predominance and mean age in the spine is 10 years and in the head is 20 years. It tends to be located in the **midline:** parasellar, fourth ventricular, or interhemispheric.

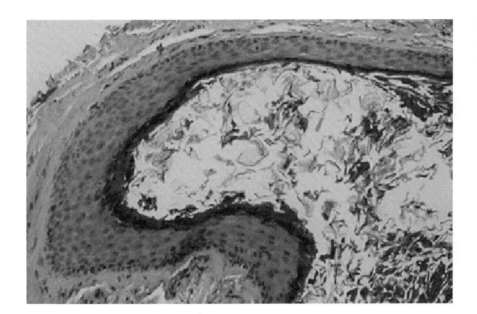

Figure 122   Epidermoid cyst (H and E). Stratified squamous epithelium around thin "dry" keratin.

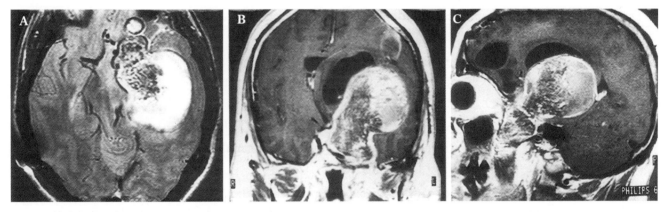

Figure 123   Dermoid tumor. T2-weighted axial (A) and T1-weighted non-infused coronal (B) and sagittal (C) MRIs demonstrating the left sided high intensity parasellar mass.

2. It appears similar to fat on MRI and has **frequent calcifications (Fig. 123)**. It is filled with oily fluid and cholesterol that causes a chemical meningitis when it leaks, and this may lead to vasospasm and death. It contains cheesy material, **pilosebaceous units** with hair shafts and sebaceous glands, sweat glands, and occasionally teeth **(Fig. 124)**. It grows by both desquamation and gland secretion and frequently ruptures.

3. Dermoid tumors may be **congenital** or acquired through trauma or lumbar puncture.

4. Dermoids (and epidermoids) rarely undergo malignant change to squamous cell carcinoma. There may be a fistula to the skin with recurrent bouts of **bacterial meningitis**.

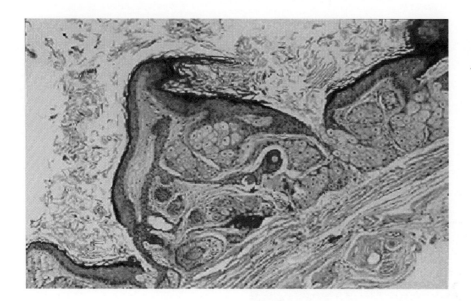

Figure 124   Dermoid cyst (H and E). Epidermis with sebaceous cysts and hair follicles.

N. Lipoma

1. It accounts for 0.2% of intracranial tumors. It presents at any age and has no sex predominance. It is usually in the **midline** (90%): above the corpus callosum, at the quadrigeminal plate, in the third ventricle, CPA, or sylvian fissure.

2. It is comprised of mature fatty tissue (**Fig. 125**). There may be peripheral **calcifications**, and it rarely contains bone, cartilage, or muscle. Fifty percent are **associated with brain malformations**.

3. Lipomas are thought to occur from maldifferentiation of the **meninx priminativa**, a mesenchyme derivative of the neural crest with both ectodermal and mesodermal tissue that forms the dura, arachnoid, and arachnoid cisterns.

4. Variants are (1) **tubulonodular**—usually anterior over the corpus callosum and associated with corpus callosal dysgenesis, cephaloceles, and frontal lobe abnormalities; and (2) **curvilinear**—usually around the splenium, and the corpus callosum tends to be normal (**Figs. 126 and 127**).

O. Chordoma

1. Mean age is 20 to 60 years and there is a **male predominance**. Forty percent occur in the **clivus** and 60% in the **sacrum** (rarely in other parts of the spine) (**Figs. 128 and 129**). They are derived from **notochord remnants** (as is the nucleus pulposus) at the extremes of the axial skeleton.

2. It is "benign" but is locally aggressive, destroys surrounding bone, and is malignant by location (usually very difficult to remove). It tends to be painful. Chordomas metastasize (25 to 40%) and may change to sarcoma.

3. Pathologically, it is lobulated, gray, soft, with sheets or cords of large vacuolated cells (**physalipherous** or bubble-bearing cells) surrounded by mucin. Immunohistochemistry is similar to the notocord with characteristics of both mesenchyme and epithelium: positive for cytokeratin and EMA (epithelial) and S100 (mesenchymal, neural crest) (**Fig. 130**).

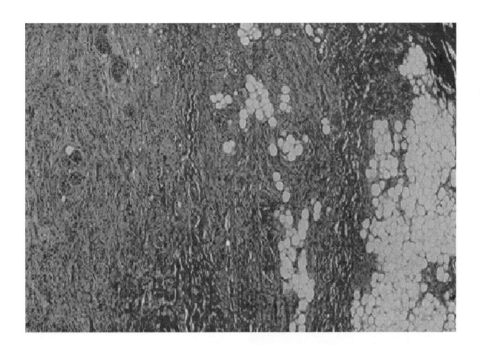

Figure 125 Intradural spinal lipoma (H and E). Adipose tissue and collagenous connective tissue infiltrating cord parenchyma.

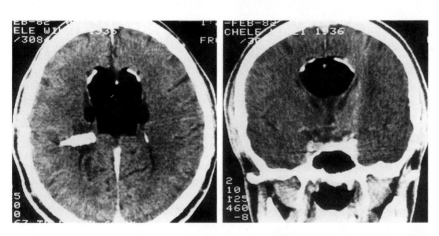

Figure 126 Corpus callosum lipoma. Non-infused axial (A) and coronal (B) CTs demonstrating a low density lesion above the corpus callosum with a rim of calcification.

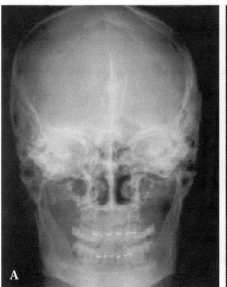
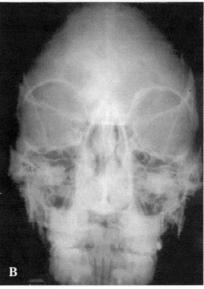

Figure 127 Corpus callosum lipoma. AP skull x-ray films demonstrate (A) curvilinear and (B) globular types of corpus callosum lipomas with calcifications.

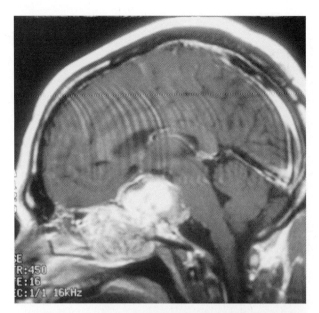

Figure 128   Clivus chordoma. Sagittal infused T1-weighted MRI demonstrating an enhancing mass eroding the clivus and filling the sella and suprasellar space.

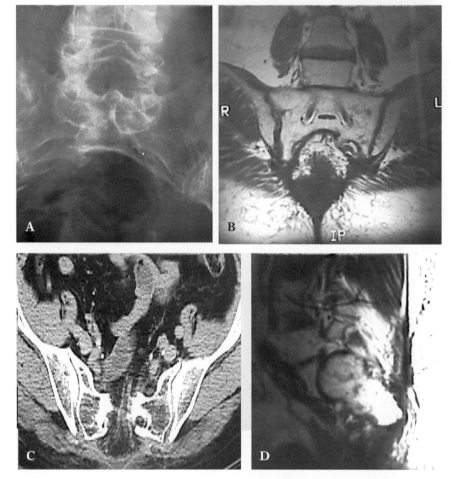

Figure 129   Sacral chordoma. AP x-ray film (A), coronal T1-weighted MRI (B), coronal CT (C), and sagittal infused T1-weighted MRI (D) demonstrating erosive lower sacral mass.

4. Chondroid chordoma—a variant that contains cartilage and has a better prognosis. Low-grade chondrosarcoma is negative for cytokeratin and EMA, but positive for S100.

5. Treatment is surgical resection and radiation. Survival is usually 5 to 7 years.

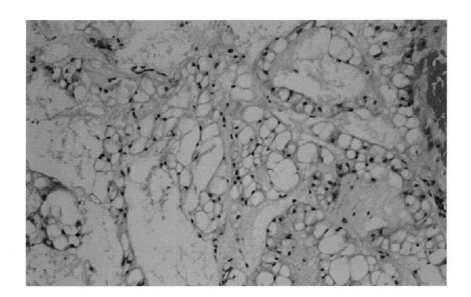

Figure 130   Chordoma (H and E). "Physaliphorus" or bubble-bearing cells in mucoid-rich stroma.

P. Glomus jugulare tumor (paraganglioma)

1. It occurs in middle age with female predominance.

2. It originates from paraganglion tissue in the adventitia of the **dome of the jugular bulb** and may produce **catecholamines**.

3. Treatment is with mastoidectomy and resection followed by radiation. They are extremely vascular and consideration should be given to preoperative embolization (**Fig. 131**).

Q. Carotid body tumor (chemodectoma)

1. It occurs at the **carotid bifurcation** and forms a painless mass below the angle of the jaw (similar to a salivary gland tumor or a branchial cleft cyst). CN IX to XII may be involved.

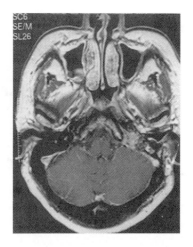

Figure 131   Glomus jugulare tumor. Infused T1-weighted axial MRI demonstrating a left-sided erhancing mass in the jugular foramen.

2. It has neurosecretory granules similar to those in the carotid body and may produce **catecholamines**.

3. Five percent are **bilateral** and 5% are malignant. There is a **familial tendency**.

4. Treatment is with surgery and/or radiation.

R. Esthesioneuroblastoma

1. It arises in the high nasal cavity from neurosecretory receptor cells or basal cells (**Fig. 132**).

2. It may metastasize to the CNS.

3. Patients are usually > 50 years.

S. Metastatic tumors to the nervous system.

1. Skull—breast, lung, and prostate carcinoma and multiple myeloma.

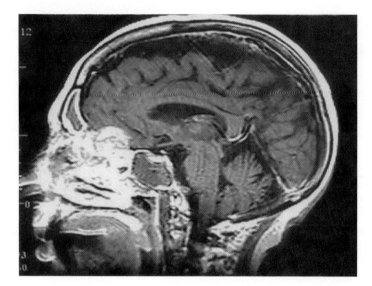

Figure 132   Esthesioneuroblastoma. Infused sagittal T1-weighted MRI demonstrating an enhancing mass invading through the floor of the anterior fossa.

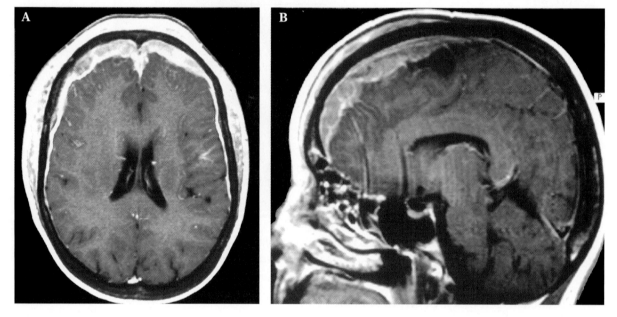

Figure 133   Leptomeningeal carcinomatosis. Axial (A), and sagittal (B) infused T1-weighted MRIs demonstrating diffuse meningeal enhancement.

2. Epidural (mainly thoracic spine)—breast, lung, and prostate carcinoma. Less frequently lymphoma, melanoma, renal cell carcinoma, multiple myeloma, and sarcoma.

3. Dural (found in 10% of diffuse metastatic case autopsies)—breast, lung, lymphoma, leukemia, melanoma, and GI tumors.

4. Leptomeningeal (found in 10% of CNS metastatic cases)—breast, lung, melanoma, and gastric carcinoma. Leptomeningeal carcinomatosis is diffuse seeding of the leptomeninges by tumor causing cranial neuropathies and CSF obstruction. The CSF has increased protein and tumor cells, decreased glucose, and no inflammatory cells (**Fig. 133**).

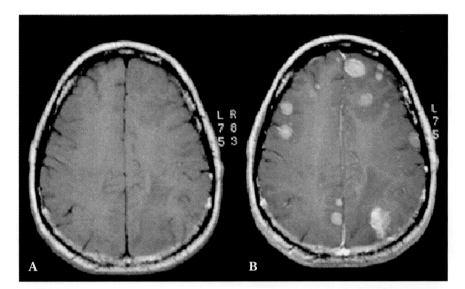

Figure 134   Multiple brain metastases. Axial noninfused (A) and infused (B) T1-weighted MRIs demonstrating the multiple enhancing lesions.

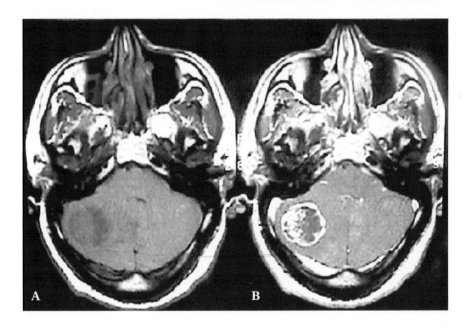

Figure 135   Cystic brain metastasis. Axial noninfused (A) and infused (B) T1-weighted MRIs demonstrating a lesion with irregular rim enhancement.

5. Parenchymal (accounts for 30% of brain tumors and mean survival is 3 to 6 months)—**lung** (35%), breast (20%), kidney (10%), melanoma (10%), and GI (5%). They are multiple in 75%. They usually occur at the **gray/white junction** and are round and **well circumscribed**. Hemorrhage is especially common with choriocarcinoma, melanoma, and renal cell carcinoma. Metastases to the spinal cord parenchyma are very rare but are usually caused by lung carcinoma and to a lesser extent breast, renal cell, and melanoma (**Figs. 134 through 137**).

T. Tumors of blood cell origin.

1. Non-Hodgkins lymphoma—usually **B cell** and diffuse. Pathologic examination demonstrates mixed small and large cells of intermediate or high grade. There is concentric **reticulin**. It is **radiosensitive**.

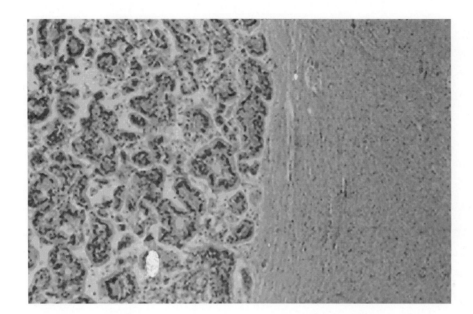

Figure 136   Metastatic carcinoma (H and E); circumscribed glandular tumor.

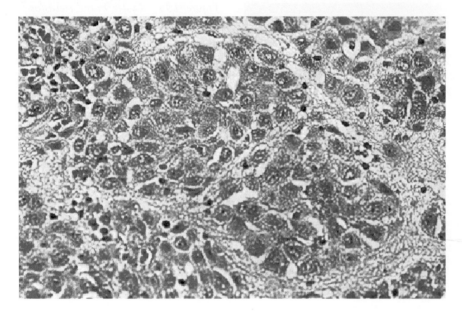

Figure 137   Melanoma (H and E); epitheliod cells with melanin inclusions.

(a) Primary CNS lymphoma—usually **parenchymal subependymal and subpial**. It is most common in **men 60 years of age who are immunocompetent and men 30 years of age who are immunosuppressed**. Risk increases with Wiskott-Aldrich syndrome, transplant patients, AIDS, collagen vascular disease, and cancer. It may be associated with disease caused by **Epstein-Barr virus** infection. They may be **hyperdense on CT** and usually enhance brightly. Thirty percent are **multiple**. Survival without treatment is < 1 year and with chemotherapy, **steroids**, and radiation is up to 3.5 years (**Figs. 138 and 139**).

(b) Secondary (metastatic) CNS lymphoma—usually intracranial **meningeal** or spinal epidural. Treat with radiation. Intravascular lymphoma is spread of lymphoma inside blood vessels, causing strokes and dementia.

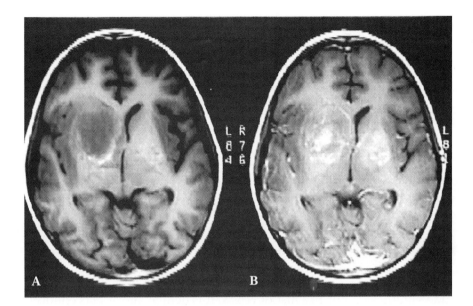

Figure 138 Primary CNS lymphoma. Axial noninfused (A) and infused (B) T1-weighted MRIs demonstrating bilateral periventricular enhancing lesions.

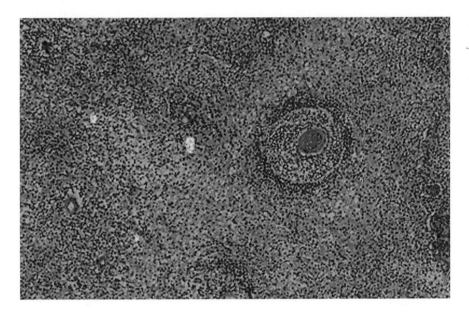

Figure 139 Lymphoma (H and E). Diffuse perivascular infiltrate with small blue cells filling the Virchow-Robin space around the vessel.

2. Hodgkin's lymphoma—has characteristic **Reed-Sternberg** binucleated cells. Varieties include lymphocyte predominant, mixed cellular, lymphocyte depleted, and nodular sclerosis. Twenty percent develop neurologic complications, usually involving the skull or meninges.

U. Plasma cell disorders

1. Plasmacytoma (single location) and multiple myeloma (**MM**) (more than one location)—locations include vertebral bodies (fractures), ribs, and skull (70% of MM, the inner table appears punched-out). Pathologic examination demonstrates mixed small and large cells of intermediate or high grade. There is concentric reticulin and Russel bodies (eosinophilic intracytoplasmic inclusions filled with immunoglobulins).

2. Waldenstrom's macroglobulinemia—plasma cells accumulate in the bone marrow, liver, spleen, and lymph nodes. There are no lytic lesions. Twenty-five percent of cases develop neurologic complications, including peripheral neuropathy, stroke, and subarachnoid hemorrhage.

3. Heavy chain disease.

4. Primary amyloidosis—accumulation of light chains.

V. Histiocytosis X (Langerhan's cell histiocytosis)—usually involves bone. Extra-skeletal sites are involved in 20%. Of these, 90% are intracranial. Symptoms include diabetes insipidus. Pathologically characterized by multinucleated giant cells. Electron microscopy demonstrates cytoplasmic Birbeck bodies that look like tennis rackets.

1. Letterer-Siwe disease—acute disseminated histiocytosis. Occurs in children ages 2 to 4 years. Death usually ensues within 2 years. It involves multiple organs.

2. **Eosinophilic granuloma**—unifocal Langhan's histiocytosis. It is benign and affects children and young adults. It is a painful, solitary, **lytic bone lesion with clear margins** (no sclerotic rim). Lesions involve the full thickness of the skull and may occasionally be located in the brain, spinal cord, or dura. Treatment is with excision or radiation.

3. Multifocal histiocytosis—chronic, recurrent, and disseminated. Onset is before 5 years. It causes respiratory infections and infiltrates lymph nodes, liver, spleen, bones, orbit, pituitary, and hypothalamus. **Hand-Schüller-Christian disease**—lytic bone lesions, exopthalamos, and diabetes insipidus.

W. Leukemia—may be diffuse or focal (solid green mass called a **chloroma**). It **hemorrhages** frequently, and this results in 50% of the deaths. It usually involves the leptomeninges (especially ALL). It is protected from chemotherapy in the CNS by the BBB. Evaluation should include a lumbar puncture, which, if positive, should be followed by prophylactic radiation and intrathecal chemotherapy with **methotrexate (MXT)**. **Necrotizing leukoencephalopathy** may develop in patients < 5 years and is due to MXT injury to the myelin after the radiation has broken down the BBB.

X. Nontumor cysts

1. Colloid cyst

(a) Mean age is 20 to 40 years and there is no sex predominance.

(b) It is normally in the **anterior roof of the third ventricle** between the columns of the fornices and is frequently attached to the stroma of the choroid.

(c) It is believed to be of **endodermal origin** from a vestigial third ventricular structure (the paraphysis) and is rarely associated with craniopharyngioma. The cyst may be pendulous and cause intermittent CSF obstruction with a ball-valve mechanism.

(d) It is filled with mucus (mucopolysaccharides) that on CT may be either hyperdense (two-thirds) or hypodense (one-third). On MRI, it is **hyperintense on T1-weighted images** and hypointense on T2-weighted images (**Figs. 140 and 141**).

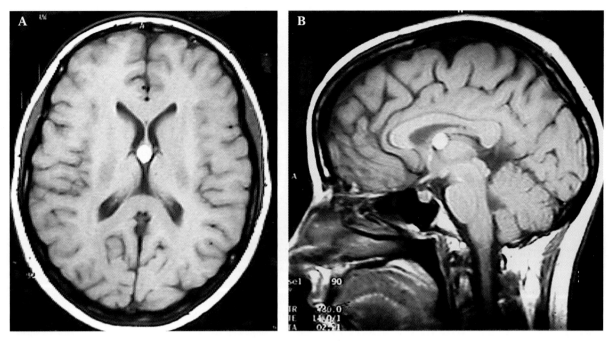

Figure 140   Colloid cyst. Axial (A) and sagittal (B) T1-weighted noninfused MRIs demonstrate hyperintense cyst in the roof of the third ventricle.

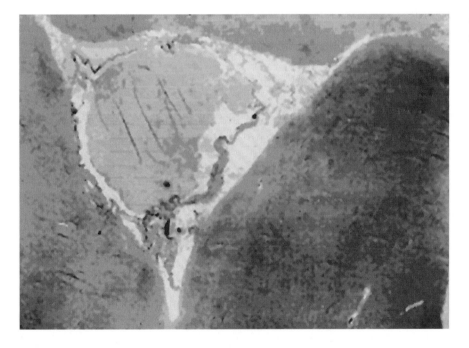

Figure 141   Colloid cyst (H and E) in the third ventricle filled with mucin.

(e) There are no calcifications and there is usually enhancement of the cyst wall. The fibrous capsule is lined by a single pseudostratified layer of columnar cells with occasional cilia and PAS-positive goblet cells. The smallest documented cyst causing death is 1 cm.

(f) Consider surgery if the cyst is >7 mm because resection is curative.

2. Arachnoid cyst—congenital, male pre-dominance, usually in children (75%), and becomes symptomatic in 70% of cases. Locations are **middle fossa** (60%), suprasellar (10%), quadrigeminal cistern (10%), posterior fossa (10%, CPA and cisterna magna), and convexity (5%). It is associated with **subdural hematomas** because of tearing of the bridging veins that traverse the cyst (**Fig. 142**).

3. Neuroepithelial cyst—caused by the infolding of developing neuroectoderm. They may be located in the ependyma, choroid plexus, and choroidal fissure.

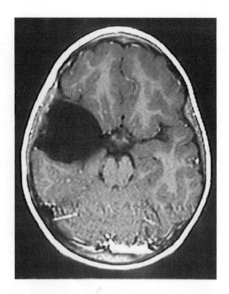

Figure 142   Arachnoid cyst. Infused T1-weighted MRI demonstrates nonenhancing middle fossa extra-axial cyst.

4. Enterogenous (neurenteric) cyst—filled with **endoderm** of GI or respiratory mucosa. They have a single layer of cuboidal/columnar cells with interspersed goblet cells. Locations are spine (80%), intracranial (15%), CPA, and craniocervical junction. There is a male predominance. They may be due to notocord-gut fusion.

5. Cavum septum pellucidum—at the level of the caudate head. CSF is in between the sheets of the septum pellucidum in the lateral ventricles.

6. Cavum vergae—a posterior continuation of the cavum septum pellucidum.

7. Cavum velum interpositum—in the third ventricle because of failure of fusion of the tela choroidea.

Y. Peripheral nerve sheath tumors

1. Traumatic neuroma—consists of a tangle of axons, Schwann cells, and fibroblasts in a collagen matrix. They are usually painful and rubbery.

2. Schwannoma

   (a) Accounts for 7% of intracranial tumors. Five percent are multiple, usually with **NF2**. It is benign, has no sex predominance, and mean age is 40 to 50 years (although onset is by 20 years with NF2). It grows slowly and **almost never undergoes malignant change**. Schwann cells are derived from the neural crest cells.

   (b) Schwannomas occur intracranially and along the spinal cord at the REZ of sensory nerves, in the head and neck, posterior mediastinum, retroperitoneum, and the **flexor surface of the extremities**.

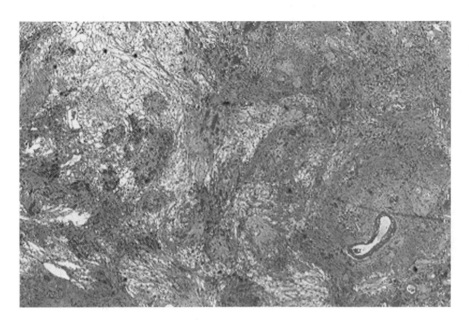

Figure 143 Schwannoma (H and E). Dense Antoni A areas with compact spindle cells, looser Antoni B areas with stellate cells.

(c) Intracranially, the most common site is on the **superior vestibular nerve** where it originates in the internal acoustic meatus at the REZ. The second most common site is the trigeminal nerve (5%), and these are located in the middle fossa (50%), both middle and posterior fossa (dumbbell, 25%), and posterior fossa (25%).

(d) Rarely, they are intra-axial in the brain or spinal cord when they form on perivascular nerves. Spinal schwannomas form on sensory nerve roots, account for 30% of spinal tumors, and may be intraspinal or dumbbell shaped.

(e) Schwannomas are firm and **encapsulated**. They are initially fusiform when intra-neural but then enlarge and become eccentric with epineurium as a capsule. They contain no axons. There is a biphasic pattern of compact **Antoni A** (fusiform cells, reticulin, and collagen) and loose **Antoni B** (stellate round cells in stroma) areas (**Fig. 143**).

(f) There are multiple different planes of fascicle groups of spindle cells that look like **schools of fish** swimming in different directions. There are **Verocay bodies**, anuclear material with pallisading cells in Antoni A areas. They are frequently **cystic**, **hemorrhagic**, and may contain fat (**Figs. 144 and 145**). Mitotic figures do not change prognosis. Immunohistochemistry is S100 positive (**Figs. 146 through 148**).

(g) Schwannomas are isointense to hypointense on T1-weighted MRI, enhance, and are rarely calcified.

(h) Variants are cellular (middle-aged females), ancient (hypocellular with cysts, calcifications, and old hemorrhage), plexiform (multinodular, not associated with NF), and melanotic (a few are malignant)

3. Neurofibroma

(a) Develops at any age and has no sex predominance. They do not occur intracranially but usually involve the posterior ganglia. They contain Schwann cells, fibroblasts, collagen,

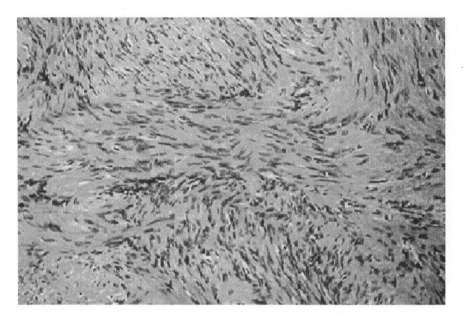

Figure 144   Schwannoma (H and E). "Schools of fish" swimming in multiple different planes.

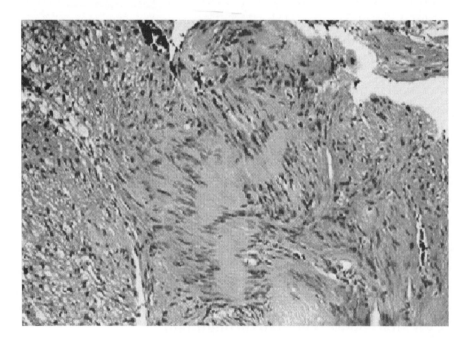

Figure 145   Schwannoma (H and E). Verocay bodies with nuclear pallisading around anuclear fibrillary material (occurs in Antoni A areas).

and reticulin. They are fusiform, **unencapsulated**, infiltrate nerves, and **rarely have cystic, fatty, or hemorrhagic changes**. Five to 13% undergo malignant change. Most are solitary cutaneous nodules coming from small terminal nerves. NF is associated with neurofibromas on larger nerve trunks and with malignant transformation (**Fig. 149**).

(b) Cutaneous neurofibroma—dermal or subcutaneous, painless, unencapsulated (so may infiltrate surrounding nerves), and soft. Multiple lesions are associated with NF1. They rarely undergo malignant transformation. Most are solitary and contain loose wavy nu-

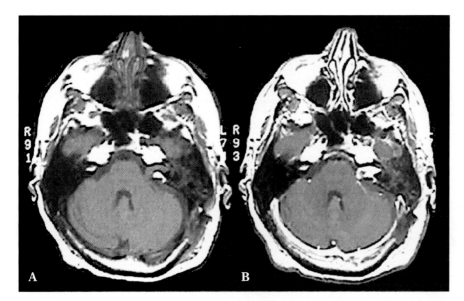

Figure 146   Vestibular schwannoma. Noninfused (A) and infused (B) axial T1-weighted MRIs demonstrating an enhancing and thickened left vestibulocochlear nerve.

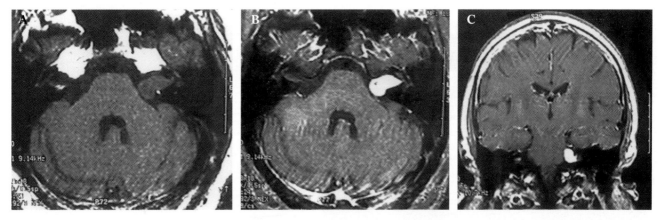

Figure 147   Vestibular schwannoma. Noninfused (A) and infused (B) axial and infused (C) coronal T1-weighted MRIs demonstrating an enhancing mass emanating from the left internal acoustic meatus.

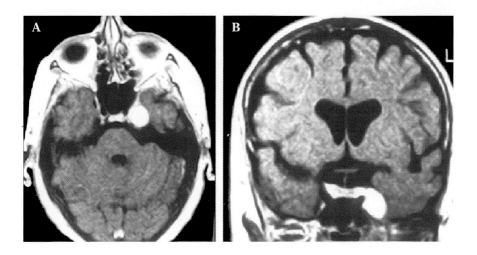

Figure 148   Trigeminal schwannoma. Axial (A) and coronal (B) infused T1-weighted MRIs demonstrating a smooth, circumscribed, enhancing mass in Meckel's cave.

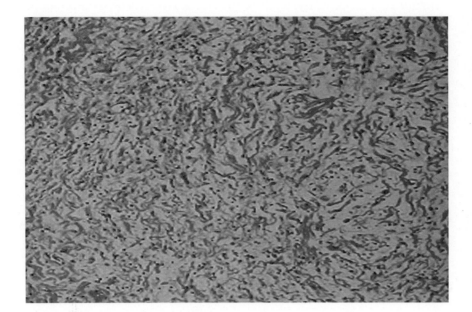

Figure 149   Neurofibroma (H and E). Elongated Schwann cells with wavy nuclei in a loose mucopolysaccharide matrix.

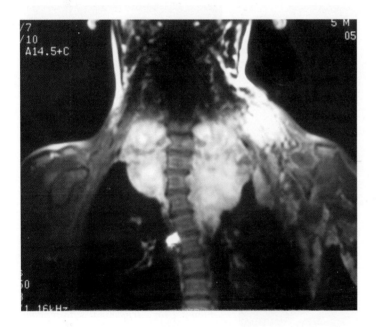

Figure 150   Plexiform neurofibroma.

clei in a matrix with axons (detected by silver stain). Immunohistochemistry is positive for vimentin, Leu7, S100, and occasionally GFAP.

(c) Intraneural neurofibroma—involves large nerve trunks, has a higher potential for malignant transformation, and is associated with NF1. The **plexiform neurofibroma** (pathognomonic of NF1) appears like an enlarged bag of worms and it may involve an entire extremity, causing elephantiasis neuromatosa. Five percent of plexiform neurofibromas undergo malignant change (**Figs. 150 and 151**).

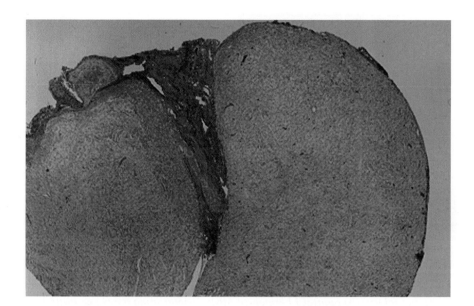

Figure 151   Plexiform neurofibroma (H and E). Diffuse enlargement of adjacent nerves.

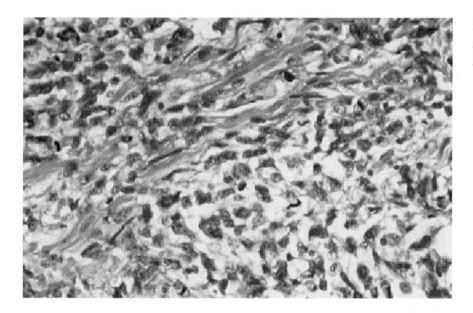

Figure 152   Malignant peripheral nerve sheath tumor (H and E). Hypercellular spindle cell neoplasm.

4. Perineuroma—rare, occurs in adolescents, involves the distal extremity, and causes a motor mononeuropathy. Pathologically, it forms an onion bulb, is made of perineural cells, and is EMA positive and S100 negative.

5. Malignant peripheral nerve sheath tumor (MPNST)—involves proximal nerves, is very painful, and has increased cellularity and mitoses with necrosis. **Fifty percent have NF1.** It very rarely develops from schwannomas. Ten percent have had prior radiation. Seventy-five percent recur and cause death. Prognosis is worse if the tumor is > 5 cm, has necrosis, or is associated with NF. Five to 13% of neurofibromas in NF1 become malignant. The most common intracranial MPNST involves the trigeminal nerve (**Fig. 152**).

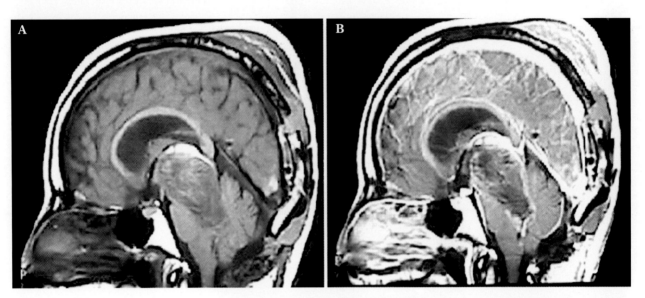

Figure 153   Pineal region GBM. Noninfused (A) and infused (B) sagittal T1-weighted MRIs demonstrating a diffuse, infiltrating, nonenhancing pineal region mass.

IX. DIFFERENTIAL DIAGNOSIS BY LOCATION

A. Pineal region—includes the suprapineal recess of the third ventricle, the **velum interpositum** (the anterior extension of the quadrigeminal cistern above the pineal gland and extending under the fornicies; may be "cavum" or filled with CSF), and the posterior commissure between the pineal gland and the colliculi. This region contains 1 to 3% of tumors and 3 to 8% of childhood tumors.

   1. Germ cell tumors—the most common tumors here (66%) with a peak age of 15 years. Germinomas (66%) are more frequent than teratomas (15%), and 5% of germinomas have a concomitant pituitary germ cell tumor (**Fig. 110**).

   2. Pineal parenchymal tumors—account for <15% (**Figs. 105 and 107**).

   3. Pineal cysts—40% of autopsy pineal masses, but only 1 to 5% of MRI pineal masses (**Fig. 108**).

   4. Others—astrocytoma (**Fig. 153**), meningioma, metastatic tumor, and vascular malformation.

B. Posterior third ventricle—meningioma, choroid plexus papilloma, and metastatic tumor.

C. Tectum—low-grade astrocytoma (detect by noticing that the inferior colliculus should always be larger than the superior colliculus).

D. Intraventricular—the septum pellucidum extends from the fornix to the corpus callosum. An absent septum pellucidum is associated with holoprosencephaly, septo-optic dysplasia, and callosal agenesis. **Cavum septum pellucidum** is present in 80% of neonates and 3% of adults. **Cavum vergae** is present in 30% of neonates and 3% of adults. These two are persistence of normal fetal cavities. Vergae is a posterior extension of the cavum septum pellucidum and never occurs without one. It is located below the corpus callosum, between the fornices, and on the next higher cut than the cavum septum pellucidum (**Fig. 154**).

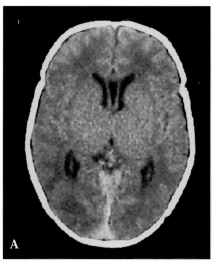 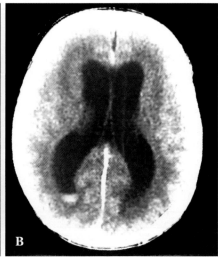

Figure 154   Cavum septum pellucidum
(A) and cavum vergae (b); noninfused CTs.

1. Primary septal tumor—astrocytoma, lymphoma, and germinoma.

2. Frontal horn/septum pellucidum tumor—central neurocytoma, giant cell astrocytoma, and subependymoma.

3. Children

    (a) Frontal horn—low-grade astrocytoma and giant cell astrocytoma.

    (b) Body—PNET and astrocytoma.

    (c) Atrium—choroid plexus papilloma, ependymoma, and astrocytoma.

    (d) Occipital and temporal horns—meningioma (rare).

    (e) Foramen of Monro—giant cell astrocytoma, colloid cyst, craniopharyngioma.

    (f) Anterior third ventricle—astrocytoma, histiocytosis (hypothalamic/infundibular), germinoma, and craniopharyngioma (extrinsic).

    (g) Fourth ventricle—pilocytic astrocytoma, medulloblastoma, ependymoma, exophytic medulla brain stem glioma, and choroid plexus papilloma.

4. Adults

    (a) Frontal horn—high-grade astrocytoma, giant cell astrocytoma, central neurocytoma, and subependymoma.

    (b) Body—astrocytoma, central neurocytoma, oligodendroglioma, and subependymoma.

    (c) Atrium—meningioma, metastatic tumor, and lymphoma.

    (d) Occipital and temporal horns—meningioma.

    (e) Foramen of Monro—high-grade astrocytoma, central neurocytoma, oligodendroglioma, subependymoma, and colloid cyst.

(f) Anterior third ventricle—colloid cyst, extrinsic pituitary tumor/aneurysm/glioma, sarcoid, and germinoma.

(g) Fourth ventricle—metastatic tumor, hemangioblastoma, exophytic brain stem glioma, and subependymoma.

5. Rarely there are choroid plexus cysts and xanthogranulomas.

E. Cerebellopontine angle (CPA) tumors—usually occur where the flocculus projects into the CPA.

1. Vestibular schwannoma (acoustic neuroma)—75%.

2. Meningioma—10%.

3. Epidermoid—5%.

4. Others—vascular lesions such as dolicoectasia, aneurysm, and AVM (2 to 5%) and metastatic tumors (1 to 2%).

5. Internal auditory canal masses—vestibular schwannoma, postoperative fibrosis, and neuritis (Bell's palsy and Ramsay-Hunt zoster otitis).

6. Temporal bone lesions involving the CPA—gradenigo's syndrome (osteomyelitis of the petrous apex with CN VI palsy, otorrhea, and retro-orbital pain), malignant external otitis, cholesteatoma (hyperintense on T1-weighted and T2-weighted MRI), and paraganglioma (slow growing, hypervascular, from the neural crest, in the cochlear promontory, and called the glomus tympanicum tumor).

F. Foramen magnum—cervicomedullary low-grade astrocytoma, anterior intradural meningioma or schwannoma, chordoma, chondroma, chondrosarcoma, and metastatic tumor. The **classic presentation** of a foramen magnum mass is progressive weakness of the ipsilateral upper limb followed in order by the ipsilateral lower limb, contralateral lower limb, and then the contralateral upper limb.

G. Sella

1. Intrasellar masses—pituitary hyperplasia (seen with puberty, pregnancy, postpartum, and end organ failure), microadenoma (< 1 cm), and nonneoplastic cyst (20% at autopsy, from the pars intermedia or Rathke's cleft). Less common are craniopharyngioma (5 to 10% are intrasellar), breast metastases, epidermoid, dermoid, and aneurysm. The pituitary gland normally enhances.

2. Suprasellar masses (SATCHMO)—"Sarcoid, pituitary adenoma, Aneurysm, Teratoma, Craniopharyngioma, Hypothalamic glioma or Hamartoma, Meningioma, and Optic glioma." In descending order of frequency: pituitary adenoma, meningioma, craniopharyngioma, hypothalamic/chiasm glioma (20 to 50% associated with NF1, enhances, hypointense on T1-weighted MRI, and usually pilocytic), and aneurysm. Less common are arachnoid cyst (10% suprasellar), Rathke's cleft cyst (rarely purely suprasellar), hypothalamic hamartoma (associated with precocious puberty, partial complex seizures, and psychologic changes, and does not enhance), sarcoid, and lymphocytic hypophysitis (anterior lobe, enhances, in peripartum women) **(Figs. 155 and 156)**.

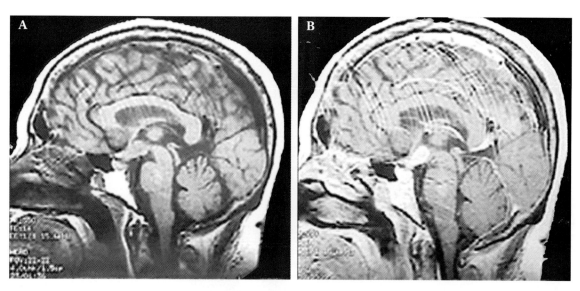

Figure 155   Neurosarcoid. Noninfused (A) and infused (B) sagittal T1-weighted MRIs demonstrate the sellar and suprasellar enhancement.

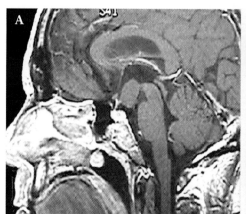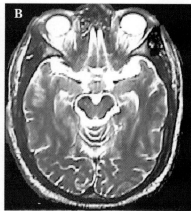

Figure 156   Hypothalamic hamartoma. Sagittal T1-weighted infused (A) and axial T2-weighted (B) MRIs demonstrating a nonenhancing mass posterior to the optic chiasm.

3. Suprasellar "hot spot" (hyperintense on T1-weighted MRI)—Rathke's cleft cyst, craniopharyngioma, subacute blood (thrombosed aneurysm, hemorrhagic tumor, and postoperatively), lipoma, dermoid, ectopic neurohypophysis, sarcoid, and histiocytosis.

4. Infundibulum—normally enhances because there is no BBB.

   (a) Children—Histiocytosis X (absent posterior pituitary bright spot and thickened stalk), germinoma, and meningitis.

   (b) Adults—sarcoid, germinoma, and metastatic tumors.

H. Skull base

   1. Anterior skull base—mucocele (forms in the sinus with obstruct of flow), inverted papilloma, osteoma (frontal sinus), rhabdomyosarcoma (most common soft tissue sarcoma in children, especially in the head and neck), squamous cell carcinoma (80% of the malignant tumors in adults), adenocarcinoma (20%), esthesioneuroblastoma (from bipolar sensory receptor cells in

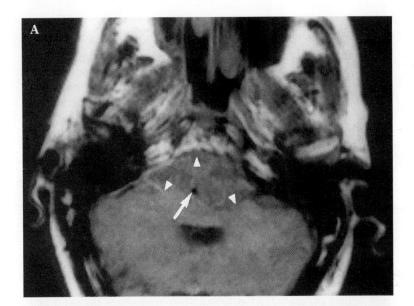

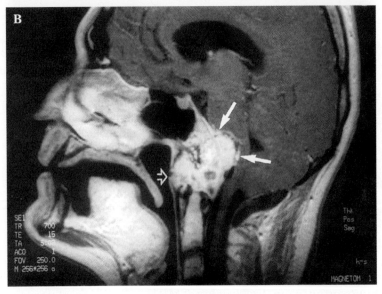

Figure 157   Clivus chondrosarcoma.T1-weighted non-infused axial (A) and infused sagittal (B) MRIs demonstrating an enhancing destructive clival mass.

the olfactory mucosa, of neural crest origin, peaks at 10 years and 40 years), encephalocele, and nasal glioma. Intrinsic lesions include fibrous dysplasia, Paget's disease, and osteopetrosis.

2. Central skull base—includes the clivus, sella, cavernous sinus, and sphenoid alae. Pituitary tumors, meningiomas, trigeminal schwannomas, juvenile angiofibroma (vascular, invasive, originates near the sphenopalatine foramen of adolescent males, most common benign nasopharyngeal tumor, and spreads along the foramen into the pterygopalatine fossa, orbit, sinus, etc.), chordoma, enchondroma (most common benign cartilaginous tumor of the skull), nasopharyngeal carcinoma, rhabdomyosarcoma, osteosarcoma (older patients, involves the maxilla or mandible, skull base involvement is rare, associated with Paget's disease and radiation), multiple myeloma, chondrosarcoma, and metastatic tumors (prostate, lung, and breast) (**Fig. 157**).

3. Posterior skull base—includes the clivus below the spheno-occipital synchondrosis and the petrous temporal bone. Clivus chordoma and metastatic tumors. A mass in the jugular foramen may be an enlarged jugular bulb, jugular vein thrombosis, paraganglioma (in the jugular bulb adventitia

Figure 158   Fibrous dysplasia; axial CT with expansion of diploe.

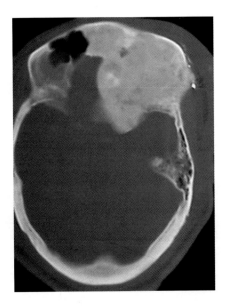

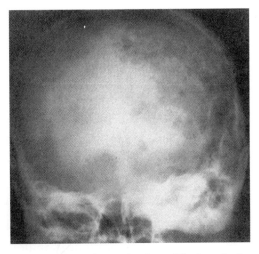

Figure 159   Fibrous dysplasia. Thickened sclerotic left orbit.

Figure 160   Fibrous dysplasia (H and E); woven bone.

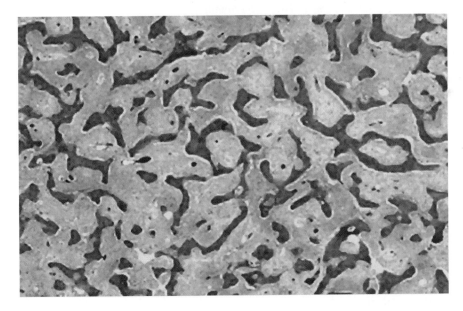

with frequent bony invasion, includes carotid body tumor, glomus jugulare, and glomus tympanicum), nasopharyngeal carcinoma metastases, schwannoma, neurofibroma, and epidermoid.

I. Diffuse skull base lesions

1. Fibrous dysplasia—presents in young adulthood. May be either mono-ostotic (70% of cases and 25% involve the skull/face) or polyostotic (30% of cases and 50% involve the skull/face). It expands and replaces normal bony medullary spaces with vascular fibrocellular tissue producing **"woven bone."** CT demonstrates thickened sclerotic bone with **"ground-glass"** expanded diploe. It is hypointense on T1-weighted images and **enhances**. There are sclerotic orbits and skull bases (facial, frontal, ethmoid, and sphenoid bones) causing **lionlike facies**. Narrowing of the optic foramen may cause visual loss. **Albright's syndrome** occurs in females and is characterized by unilateral polyostotic disease, pigmented skin lesions, and precocious puberty (**Figs. 158 through 160**).

2. Paget's disease—onset is usually after 40 years, male predominance, and it may be monoostotic or polyostotic. Early in the course, it causes destruction, whereas late in the course it causes sclerosis. There is **bony expansion** that causes symptoms by cranial nerve compression, basilar invagination, and hydrocephalus. There may be a sarcomatous degeneration, especially to osteosarcoma.

3. Langerhan's cell histiocytosis—monostotic (eosinophilic granuloma, 5 to 15 years, involves the skull) or diffuse (in young to middle age).

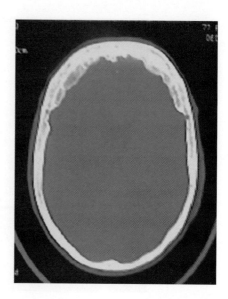

Figure 161   Hyperostalis frontalis interna. Axial CT bone window demonstrates irregular thickening of the inner table of the frontal bone.

J. General calvarial thickening—normal variant, phenytoin (Dilantin), shunted hydrocephalus, acromegaly, Paget's disease, fibrous dysplasia, sickle cell disease, and iron deficiency.

K. Regional/focal calvarial thickening—hyperostosis frontalis interna (frontal bone, elderly women, spares the superior sagittal sinus), Paget's disease, fibrous dysplasia, metastatic tumors (prostate and breast), neuroblastoma ("hair-on-end" appearance), and meningioma (**Fig. 161**).

L. Generalized thinning—normal variant, hydrocephalus, osteogenesis imperfecta, Down syndrome, lacunar skull (associated with Chiari II malformation), Cushing's disease, hyperparathyroidism, and hypophosphatemia. Craniolacunia (**Lukenschadel**) is a honeycomb pattern that is congenital and associated with spinal meningocele and myelomeningocele. It may be due to increased ICP in utero.

M. Focal thinning—**parietal foramina** (bilateral, inner and outer tables meet, no clinical significance), venous lakes, pacchionian granulations, leptomeningeal cyst, arachnoid cyst, and tumor (**Fig. 162**).

N. Holes in the skull—cephalocele, dermoid, cleidocranial dysostosis, intradiploic arachnoid cyst, NF1 (absent sphenoid wing and lambdoid suture defects), hemangioma (spoke-wheel pattern and well circumscribed), epidermoid (sclerotic rim, scalloped margins, lucent, hypointense on T1-weighted and hyperintense on T2-weighted MRI), eosinophilic granuloma (nonsclerotic and has beveled edges with uneven involvement of the inner and outer tables), Paget's disease lytic phase, multiple myeloma, and growing skull fracture (**Figs. 163 through 170**).

O. Meninges— the outer layer of dura (the periosteal layer) contains fibroblasts and blood vessels, and it does not extend caudal to the foramen magnum. The inner layer contains epithelial cells and is continuous with the spinal dura (one layer). The dura enhances a little because it has no BBB. The enhancement is patchy, smooth, thin, and most prominent near the vertex. The pia has an outer layer of collagen and inner layer of elastic fibers. **Virchow-Robin spaces** are made by the pia and CSF that

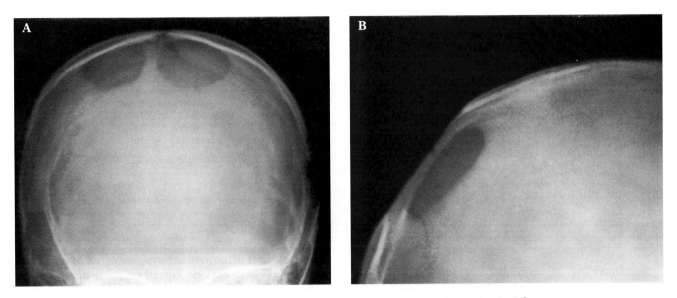

Figure 162   Parietal foramina. (A) AP and (B) lateral x-rays demonstrate the bilateral smooth-edged foramen.

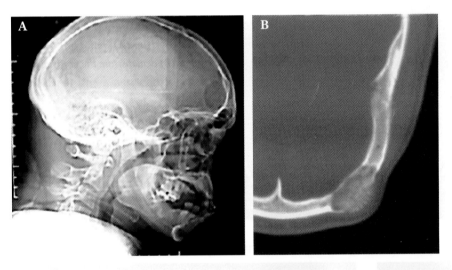

Figure 163   Hemangioma. Lateral skull x-ray film (A) and axial CT bone window (B) demonstrate the "sunburst" lesion.

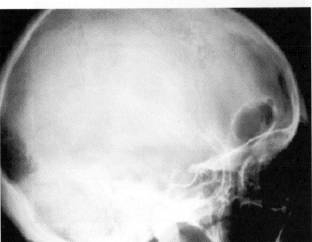

Figure 164   Epidermoid. Lateral skull x-ray film demonstrates the sclerotic margins and scalloped bone edge.

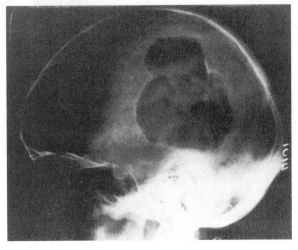

Figure 165   Skull epidermoid. Lateral skull x-ray with scalloped bone edge.

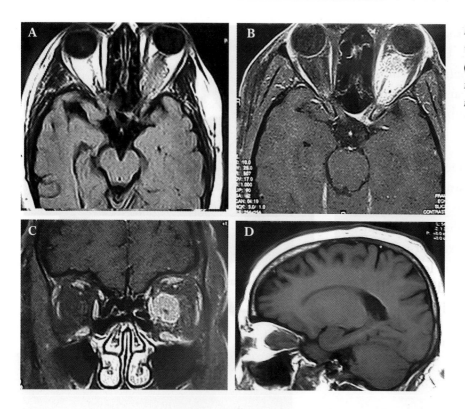

Figure 172   Optic nerve meningioma. T1-weighted axial noninfused (A) and infused (B), coronal infused (C), and sagittal non-infused (D) MRIs demonstrating enhancing mass with central hypointensity.

X. PHAKOMATOSES (NEUROCUTANEOUS DISEASES)

A. Phakomatoses—a combination of malformative, dysplastic, and neoplastic lesions of the skin and nervous system. They may be hereditary or occur sporadically. All the more common varieties have dominant transmission except Sturge-Weber disease. There are approximately 20 types. A phakoma is tumor-like retinal lesion.

B. Neurofibromatosis type 1 (NF1)

1. **Von Recklinghausen's** neurofibromatosis, **peripheral form**, accounts for **90% of NF**, occurs in 1 in 3000 births, **autosomal dominant** transmission with 100% penetrance but variable expressivity, and located on **chromosome 17. Fifty percent occur by spontaneous mutation** without a family history. It usually has an early onset and affects mainly Caucasians. Twenty percent of cases develop CNS lesions. Thirty-three percent have mental retardation. It is cosmetically disfiguring. **Five percent develop malignant peripheral nerve sheath tumors** (MPNSTs), usually after 10 years.

2. Inclusion criteria are at least two of the following: six **café au lait spots,** two neurofibromas, **one plexiform neurofibroma,** axillary or inguinal freckling, an osseous lesion (**sphenoid dysplasia** or thinning of long bones or cortex), an **optic glioma, two Lisch nodules** (iris harmartomas, only seen with NF1) (**Fig. 173**), and a relative with NF1.

3. Associated tumors—**optic gliomas** (20% may be aggressive and they may spread along the optic radiations), low-grade astrocytomas, ependymomas, hamartomas (in the white matter and basal ganglia, no enhancement, no mass effect, and decreases with age), rare unilateral vestibu-

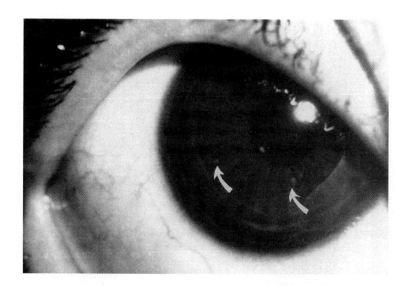

Figure 173   Lisch nodule.

lar neuromas and meningiomas, and rare spinal hamartomas and **astrocytomas**. Malignancies (2 to 5%) include MPNST, **pheochromocytoma**, and leukemia.

4. Neurofibromas develop on the posterior nerve roots and may be completely intradural (20%) or dumbbell (15%).

5. Other associated conditions—**scoliosis**, widened spinal canal, **posterior vertebral body scalloping** (by dural ectasias), patulous dura, meningocele, renal artery stenosis, aqueductal stenosis (by ependymal granulations), seizures, microphthalmoa, retinal phakomas, **moyamoya-type arterial occlusions**, aneurysms, AVMs, mental retardation (5%), and learning disability (40%) (**Fig. 174**).

C. Neurofibromatosis type 2 (NF2)

1. **Central form** occurs in 1 in 135,000 births, **autosomal dominant** transmission, located on **chromosome 22**, and has a later onset.

2. Associated tumors—**bilateral vestibular schwannomas, meningiomas, astrocytomas**, hamartomas, **spinal ependymomas** (spinal astrocytomas are more common in NF1), and nerve root schwannomas. There are less café au lait spots, cutaneous neurofibromas (more likely to be schwannomas), and plexiform neurofibromas. There are no Lisch nodules.

3. Inclusion criteria—bilateral vestibular schwannoma or a relative with NF2 and one vestibular schwannoma or two of the following: neurofibroma, meningioma, glioma, schwannoma, or postcapsular cataract at a young age. Twenty percent have spinal nerve schwannomas (70% are intradural extramedullary, 15% are extradural, and 15% are dumbbell). Two to 10% of people with a vestibular schwannoma have NF2. The osseous changes are caused by tumors, not dural ectasias (**Fig. 175**).

D. Neurofibromatosis type 5—segmental, confined to one part of the body.

E. Tuberous sclerosis (TS)

1. **Bourneville's disease, autosomal dominant** transmission, usually sporadic (there are frequent forme-frustes), possibly located on chromosomes 9 and 11, and occurs in 1 in 10,000 to

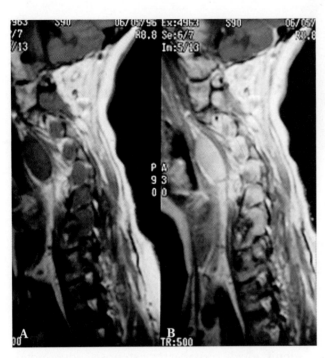

Figure 174   NF1. Sagittal T1-weighted noninfused (A) and infused (B) MRIs with multiple enhancing thickened nerve roots.

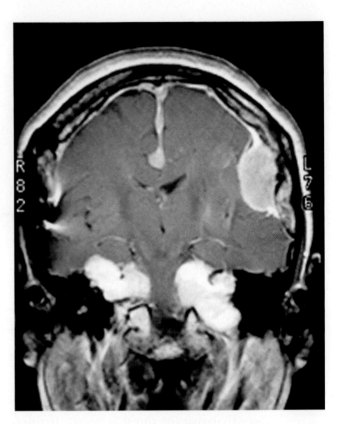

Figure 175   NF2. Infused coronal T1-weighted MRI with bilateral vestibular schwannomas and meningiomas.

100,000 births. It may be diagnosed by a facial angiofibroma, peri-ungal and subungal fibroma, or fibrous plaque of the forehead or scalp. The classic triad occurs in < 50% of cases and includes mental retardation (two-thirds) seizures, and **adenoma sebaceum** (angiofibromas).

2. Associated tumors

    (a) Tubers (seen in 95% of cases)—multiple firm lesions that are hamartomas with large dysplastic neurons and astrocytes in the thalamostriate sulcus, cortex, and subependymal region. These cause **candle guttering** in the floor of the lateral ventricle, frequently calcify, and **occasionally enhance**.

    (b) **Subependymal giant cell astrocytoma** (15% of cases)—located near the foramen of Monro, rarely undergoes malignant change, grows slowly, and enhances.

    (c) Cardiac rhabdomyoma (30% of cases)

    (d) Renal angiomyolipoma (60% of cases)

    (e) Cysts in the lung, liver, and spleen

    (f) Pancreatic adenoma

    (g) Retinal harmartoma (> 50% of cases)—rarely affects vision.

3. Associated conditions—hydrocephalus (25%), moyamoya changes of cerebral vessels, thoraco-abdominal aortic aneurysm, **ash-leaf** hypopigmented macules, **shagreen patches** (subepidermal orange peel fibrosis of the lower trunk), and cystic metacarpals. The first symptoms may

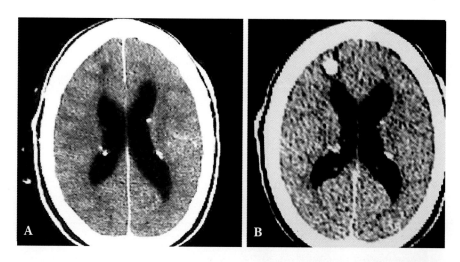

Figure 176   Tuberous sclerosis. Noninfused (A) and infused (B) axial CTs demonstrate multiple calcified tubers lining the lateral ventricles ("candle guttering") and an enhancing right frontal tuber.

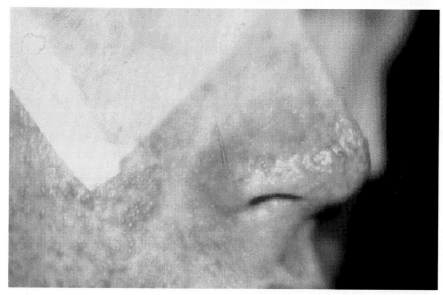

Figure 177   Adenoma sebaceum. Facial lesion with TS.

be **"salaam" spasms** of flexion myoclonus that can be treated with ACTH. Ninety percent develop skin lesions (usually ash-leaf spots) by 10 years of age. There are frequent behavioral problems (hyperkinetic or aggressive) (**Figs. 176 and 177**).

F. Von Hippel–Lindau syndrome (VHL)

   1. **Autosomal dominant** transmission, located on **chromosome 3**, and occurs in 1 in 40,000 births. It rarely presents before 20 years and renal cell carcinoma usually occurs near 40 years. Twenty percent of hemangioblastomas are in patients with VHL. The cerebellar hemangioblastoma is Lindau's tumor. A cerebellar hemangioblastoma with an extra CNS lesion is Lindau's disease. A retinal hemangioma is von Hippel's tumor.

   2. Associated tumors

      (a) **Hemangioblastomas** (seen in 60% of cases): Cerebellum (65%), brain stem (20%), and spinal cord (15%).

      (b) **Retinal hemangiomas** (50% of cases)

      (c) **Renal cell carcinoma** (30% of cases) and angiomatosis

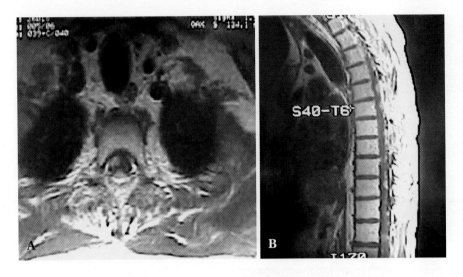

Figure 178   Von Hippel-Lindau syndrome. Infused axial (A) and sagittal (B) T1-weighted thoracic MRIs demonstrating multiple superficial parenchymal enhancing lesions.

     (d) **Pheochromocytoma** (10% of cases).

     (e) Cysts (60% of cases)—liver, pancreas, and kidney.

     (f) Epididymal cystadenoma.

   3. Diagnosis—based on multiple CNS hemangioblastomas or one CNS hemangioblastoma and one visceral lesion with a first-order relative with VHL (**Figs. 178 and 179**).

G. Sturge-Weber disease—there is **no obvious genetic transmission**. It is characterized by a port-wine stain (**facial nevus flammeus**, often in the distribution of the first division of the trigeminal nerve) and ipsilateral **venous angioma of the leptomeninges** (enhances), choroid of the eye, or choroid plexus. There are intracortical (especially parieto-occipital) **tram-track calcifications** that develop after 2 years. There is **atrophy** of a hemisphere, seizures, mental retardation, hemiparesis, hemisensory loss, homonymous hemianopsia, glaucoma (20%), ipsilateral calvarial thickening, large frontal sinus, and prominent subependymal veins. The congestion in the cortical draining veins are believed to cause stasis, hypoxia, progressive atrophy, and dystrophic calcifications in the **middle layers of the cortical gray matter** (Fig. 180).

H. Rendu-Osler-Weber syndrome (ROW)—**hereditary hemorrhagic telangiectasia**, **autosomal dominant transmission**, and characterized by multiple mucocutaneous telangiectasias (in the skin, GI, and GU tracts), visceral vascular malformations (AVMs of the liver, lung, brain, and spinal cord), and aneurysms. Fifty percent of brain symptoms are due to pulmonary AV-fistulas with **paradoxical emboli and abscesses**. There is increased risk of thrombosis as a result of polycythemia. Other symptoms include hepatic encephalopathy, GU hemorrhage, GI hemorrhage, and **epistaxis** (85%). The fragile vessels bleed easily and the red spiderlike lesions blanch with pressure. One-third of patients with multiple AVM's have ROW or Wyburn-Mason syndrome.

I. Wyburn-Mason syndrome—unilateral cutaneous vascular nevi of the face and trunk with retinal, optic nerve, visual pathway, and midbrain AVMs.

J. Ataxia-telangiectasia—oculocutaneous telangiectasias and cerebellar ataxia (caused by anterior vermian atrophy). There is a defect in DNA repair, transmission is autosomal recessive, and symptoms begin in childhood. It is associated with an increase in infections and cancer, and death usually occurs by 20 years.

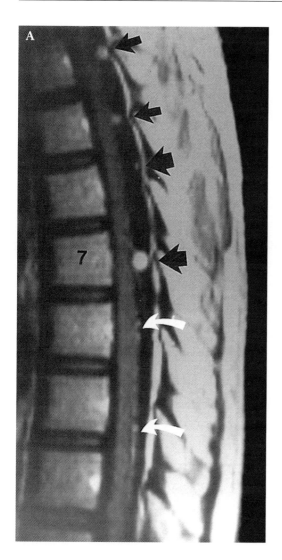

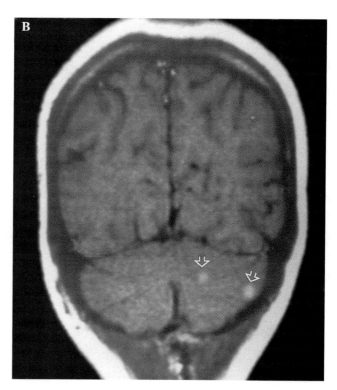

Figure 179   Von Hippel-Lindau syndrome. Infused sagittal T1-weighted MRI of the thoracic spine (A) demonstrating multiple enhancing dorsal masses. Coronal T1-weighted infused MRI of brain (B) demonstrating two enhancing cerebellar hemangioblastomas.

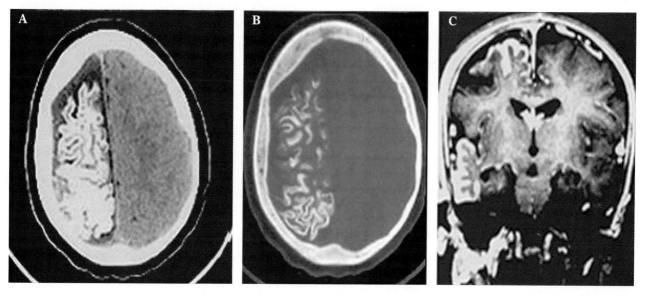

Figure 180   Sturge-Weber syndrome. Axial CT (A) and bone window (B) demonstrate the "tram track" cortical calcifications and hemispheric atrophy, and coronal infused T1-weighted MRI (C) with enhancing cortical venous malformations and hemiatrophy.

K. Klippel-Trenaunay-Weber syndrome—angio-osteohypertrophy (overgrowth of vessels and bones). One limb is usually enlarged. It is associated with leptomeningeal AVMs (some spinal) and dermatomal cutaneous hemangiomas.

L. Epidermal nevus syndrome—ipsilateral nevus and bone thickening associated with mental retardation, seizures, hemiparesis, and gyral malformations.

XI. INTOXICATIONS AND DRUGS

A. Carbon monoxide—hemoglobin binds carbon monoxide 250 times more avidly than it does O_2. Carbon monoxide also impedes oxygen release. When the hemoglobin is 25% saturated with carbon monoxide (carboxyhemoglobin), the patient may develop headaches, at 45% confusion, at 55% seizures and coma, and >70% death from dysrhythmia. A cherry-red brain develops with **bilateral GPm necrosis (Figs. 181 and 182)**.

B. Cyanide—binds cytochrome oxidase and halts cellular respiration. This leads to cerebral edema, SAH, respiratory failure, seizures, and death.

C. Ethanol (ETOH)

   1. Chronic use—associated with infections, peripheral neuropathy, strokes, cerebral atrophy (especially white matter), and ventricular enlargement. The changes may be caused by a direct toxic effect or by associated nutritional deficits (possibly thiamin). ETOH cerebellar degeneration involves the **superior vermis** and causes leg ataxia with a wide-based gait. ETOH use is associated with central pontine myelinolysis (CPM), Wernicke-Korsakoff syndrome (see section XIV), cardiomyopathy, myopathy, and Marchiafava-Bignami disease.

   2. A serum ETOH level >450 mg/dL is usually lethal unless there is substantial tolerance.

   3. ETOH withdrawal—tremulousness (1 to 2 days), hallucinations/illusions (1 to 2 days), seizures (24 hours), and delirium tremens (2 to 4 days, 5 to 15% fatal, confusion, delusions, hallucinations, tremor, sleeplessness, and autonomic overactivity with tachycardia, hyperthermia, increased sweating, and mydriasis). Treat withdrawal with chlordiazepoxide (Librium) or diazepam (Valium).

D. Fetal alcohol syndrome

   1. The world's leading cause of mental retardation and birth defects. The fetus is most susceptible shortly after conception and high levels in the first 2 months may be teratogenic.

   2. Manifestations

      (a) CNS dysfunction—mental retardation, seizures, decreased white matter, periventricular heterotopias, hypotonicity, and cerebellar dysfunction.

      (b) Craniofacial deformities—short palpebral fissures, epicanthal folds, low nasal bridge, short upturned nose, cleft palate, hypoplastic upper lip, and microcephaly.

      (c) Short body and decreased postnatal growth.

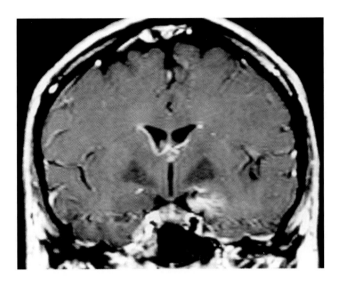

Figure 181   Carbon monoxide toxicity. Coronal T1-weighted MRI with bilateral hypointense GPs.

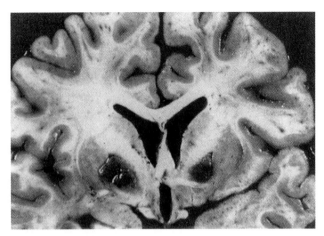

Figure 182   Carbon monoxide poisoning. Gross specimen demonstrating bilateral hemorragic necrosis of the globus pallidus.

E. Methanol—a potential contaminant in homemade liquor such as "moonshine." It is converted by ETOH dehydrogenase to formaldehyde and formic acid (blocks cellular respiration). It causes necrosis of the lateral putamen and claustrum, optic disc swelling (caused by ischemia at the watershed zone between the CNS and the optic blood supply), edema, acidosis, nausea, and vomiting. **Blindness** may develop after ingestion of 4 mL and death after ingestion of 100 mL.

F. Ethylene glycol—antifreeze. It is converted to glycoaldehyde and glycolic acid, and causes edema, Ca^{++} oxylate crystal deposition in the blood vessels, and acidosis. Ingestion of 100 mL may be lethal.

G. Isopropyl alcohol—rubbing alcohol, does not cause acidosis. Ingestion of 250 mL is lethal.

H. Hexachlorophene—germicide. It is absorbed through the skin and when exposure is significant causes spongiform degeneration of white matter.

I. Dilantin—causes **atrophy of the Purkinje and granular cell layers of the cerebellum**. It also causes **congenital fetal hydantoin syndrome** with growth retardation, mental retardation, craniofacial deformities, limb deformities, microcephaly, hydrocephalus, and neural tube defects.

J. Opiates—cause hypothermia, decreased respiration, miosis, constipation, urinary retention, pruritus, and sphincter of Oddi spasm (pancreatitis). Treat overdose with naloxone (Narcan) 0.7 mg/70 kg IV q2h. Withdrawal may occur after 16 hours with rhinorrhea, lacrimation, sweating, insomnia, mydriasis, twitches, and cold/hot flashes, after 36 hours with diarrhea, and peaks at 72 hours. It is usually only potentially fatal in infants. Withdrawal can be treated with methadone, 10 to 20mg BID, a narcotic with less euphoria and less production of desire for more narcotics.

K. Barbiturates

1. They may increase GABA levels are metabolized in the liver and excreted from the kidney.

2. They cause decreased mental status, respiratory rate, blood pressure, temperature, DTRs, and pupillary reactivity. Chronic use causes dysarthria, nystagmus, and incoordination. Severe intoxication causes slow and shallow respirations, coma, pulmonary edema, retention of mild pupillary reflexes, decreased brain stem reflexes, and a flat EEG.

3. Clearance is proportional to urine output and may be increased by fluid boluses. Bicarbonate increases excretion of phenobarbital only. Dialysis may be necessary.

4. Withdrawal may occur in 12 to 72 hours with insomnia, hypotension, tremor, seizures, REM rebound, and death. Treat with phenobarbital 0.5 g IM and attempt to wean over 14 to 21 days.

L. Benzodiazepines—safer, less addictive, less respiratory suppression, less hypotension, and less hypnotic than barbiturates. They bind GABA receptors to increase Cl⁻ influx for postsynaptic inhibition, and affect the cortex (decreases seizures) and the limbic system (decreases anxiety).

M. Antipsychotic medications—neuroleptics and psychotropics. They block postsynaptic dopaminergic D1 and D2 receptors. The D2 receptors are in the frontal cortex, hippocampus, and limbic system. The D1 receptors are in the striatum and blockage causes Parkinson-like side effects and increased PR.

1. Phenothiazines—chlorpromazine (Thorazine) and prochlorperazine (Compazine) have antiemetic, antihistamine, and antischizophrenic activities. Side effects include:

(a) Parkinsonian side effects that develop within 3 weeks. Treatment is with anticholinergics.

(b) Dystonia of the face and tongue, torticollis, and dyskinesia (tonic spasm of limbs) that develops early. Treatment is with dipherylhydramine (Benadryl) or amantadine.

(c) Akathisia/restlessness treated with propranolol.

(d) **Tardive dyskinesia** (dystonic movements of the limbs and trunk) that develops late. It occurs by hypersensitivity to dopamine in the basal ganglia or decreased GABA.

(e) Neuroleptic malignant syndrome—hyperthermia, increased serum CK, autonomic instability, rigidity, stupor, and catatonia. It is most common with haloperidal (Haldol) and fluphenazine. Mortality is 20%. It occurs from blockage of DA receptors in the basal ganglia and hypothalamus. Treatment is with dantrolene or bromocriptine.

(f) Cholestatic jaundice, agranulocytosis, seizures, orthostatic hypotension, and mental status changes.

2. Butyrophenones—haloperidal (Haldol) has similar side effects to phenothiazines but without any anti-adrenergic action and is also used to treat **Tourette's syndrome** and **Huntington's disease**.

N. Marchiafava-Bignami disease—rare, demyelination and necrosis of the **genu and body of the corpus callosum**. It was first described in Italian men drinking cheap red wine.

O. Central pontine myelinolysis (CPM)—occurs with rapid correction of hyponatremia. It is probably an osmotic injury to the vascular endothelium that disrupts the BBB and causes edema. It affects oligodendrocytes **where gray matter is interspersed with white matter** (mainly in the pons). Pathologic examination reveals **demyelination and necrosis with preserved axons and neurons and absence of inflammatory cells. (Figs. 183 and 184)**.

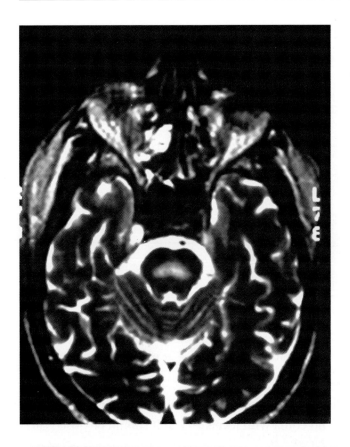

Figure 183   Central pontine myelinolysis. Axial T2-weighted MRI with central pontine hyperintensity.

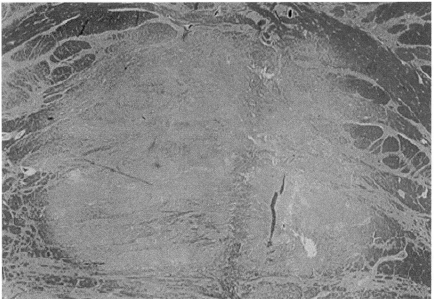

Figure 184   Central pontine myelinolysis (LFB). Central demyelination with rim of preserved myelin.

P. Antidepressants

1. Monoamine oxidase inhibitors—increase NE, 5-HT, and EPI levels and increase NE release. They increase heart rate (HR) and blood pressure (BP). Side effects include hypertension, especially with phenothiazines, stimulants, tricyclic antidepressants, tyramine, cheese, red wine, and beer.

2. Tricyclic antidepressants—**decrease the re-uptake** of amines and thus increase the levels of NE and 5-HT, and decrease ACh (urinary retention and orthostatic hypotension). Side effects

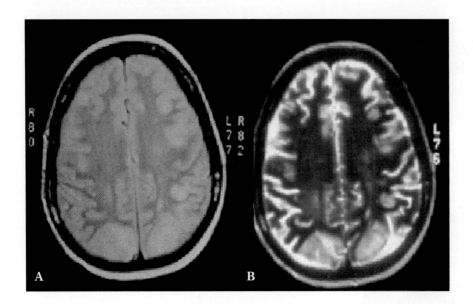

Figure 185   Methotrexate toxicity. Axial proton density (A) and T2-weighted (B) MRIs demonstrate the bilateral symmetric demyelinating lesions.

include insomnia and agitation that can be treated with phenothiazine at night. These should not be taken with MAO inhibitors.

    3. Lithium—used to treat bipolar disease. Side effects include nephrogenic diabetes insipidus and asterixis; overdose causes ataxia, nystagmus, and coma with levels > 3.5. It should be dosed carefully with renal insufficiency or thiazides.

Q. Stimulants

    1. Amphetamines (analeptics)—increase respiratory rate and BP and decrease appetite. They are used to treat children with attention deficit disorder, fatigue, obesity, and narcolepsy. Intoxication causes hallucinations, SAH, and vasculitis.

    2. Methylphenidate (Ritalin)—used to treat narcolepsy and children with attention deficit disorder.

    3. Caffeine—causes hyperglycemia, diuresis, and cardiac stimulation.

XII. CHEMOTHERAPY

A. Methotrexate—folic acid antagonist. It can cause meningitis, encephalitis, transverse myelitis, stroke, **subacute necrotizing leukoencephalitis** (with coagulation necrosis, lipid-laden macrophages, absence of inflammatory cells, mineralizing angiopathy of the gray matter, and mainly affects astrocytes) that is seen when used with radiation (**Fig. 185**).

B. Cisplatin—causes neurosensory hearing loss, visual loss, leukoencephalopathy, and sensory and autonomic neuropathy involving axons and myelin.

C. Vincristine—used to treat lymphoma and leukemia, impairs **microtubule formation**, and causes axonal degeneration with peripheral neuropathy. The blood-brain barrier (BBB) spares CNS of vincristine's effects, but it is lethal by respiratory failure if injected intrathecally.

D. Nitrosurea (BCNU)—associated with necrotizing encephalomyelopathy with arterial obliteration and axonal swelling if given arterially. Directly implanted in the tumor bed to treat GBM.

E. Procarbazine—used to treat malignant gliomas, pulmonary carcinoma, and Hodgkin's disease; causes mood changes.

XIII. METAL TOXICITIES

A. Arsenic—from insecticides. It causes encephalopathy, peripheral neuropathy, abdominal pain, nausea and vomiting, diarrhea, and shock. Chronic exposure causes malaise, **Mee's transverse white lines on the fingernails** and increased pigment and hyperkeratosis on the palms and soles. It can be **detected in hair** and urine. Treatment is with **BAL**.

B. Lead (plumbism)—causes encephalitis in children (pica from paint ingestion) that manifests as irritability, seizures, abdominal pain, ataxia, coma, and increased ICP. In adults, it causes pure motor demyelinating peripheral neuropathy (especially the radial nerve with wristdrop), anemia, and a **gingival lead line**. Diagnosis is by RBC basophilic stippling, long bone metaphyseal lead lines, increased serum lead levels, and **increased urinary copropophyrin and $_\delta$-aminolevulinic acid**. Treatment is with **EDTA, BAL, and penicillamine**.

C. Mercury—from contaminated fish ingestion and exposure to felt hat dyes. It causes psychologic dysfunction (**"mad as a hatter"**), **tremor**, **movement disorders**, peripheral neuropathy, cerebellar signs, GI dysfunction, and renal tubular necrosis. Treatment is with **penicillamine**. BAL actually increases mercury levels in the brain.

D. Manganese—occurs in miners. It causes **parkinsonian symptoms**, psychologic disorders, and headache. There is neuronal loss and gliosis in the pallidum and striatum. The symptoms are improved with L-DOPA. Chelator medications do not help.

XIV. VITAMIN DEFICIENCIES

A. Thiamin deficiency

1. It is common with chronic alcoholics, GI tumors, dialysis, intravenous feedings, and gastric plication. Thiamin is needed as a cofactor for some enzymes, especially those involved in carbohydrate metabolism. The mamillary bodies, which are frequently affected, have the highest transketolase activity in the normal brain. There may be abnormal release of excitatory neurotransmitters in Wernicke's encephalopathy and decreased serotonin in Korsakoff's psychosis. Deficiency is more frequent in Europe because of hereditary thiamin binding to transketolase.

2. Wernicke's encephalopathy

   (a) Signs include **conjugate gaze and lateral rectus palsies, nystagmus, gait ataxia, and confusion**. Rarely it may lead to coma, hypotension, and hypothermia.

   (b) It affects the **mamillary bodies**, **periventricular** thalamus and hypothalamus, **periaqueductal gray**, floor of the fourth ventricle (dorsal motor nuclei of X and the vestibular nuclei), and superior cerebellar vermis. The gaze palsies are related to CN

III and VI nuclei lesions, nystagmus to vestibular nuclei lesions, and ataxia to superior cerebellar vermian lesions.

(c) It involves both the gray and white matter, causing a brown-gray discoloration, edema, hemorrhage, demyelination, necrosis, loss of Purkinje's cells, and reactive astrocytosis.

(d) Laboratory findings include increased pyruvate and TTP and decreased transketolase.

(e) Mortality is 17% and is usually due to infection or associated cirrhosis. Treatment is with thiamin 50 mg IV and then 50 mg IM qd, until normal diet is resumed. Ocular movements recover first, and horizontal nystagmus and ataxia tend to persist longer.

3. Korsakoff's psychosis—a more chronic disorder characterized by deterioration in **short-term memory and learning** with sparing of immediate memory. There is frequently unintentional confabulation by poor memory of recent events. It is usually associated with Wernicke's encephalopathy. Lesions are in the **MD thalamus**. HSV or tumors involving the inferomedial temporal lobe may also cause a similar syndrome. Complete recovery occurs in 20% of patients.

4. Beriberi—most common in rice eaters. It causes peripheral neuropathy with axonal degeneration and demyelination, autonomic dysfunction (orthostatic hypotension), and rarely heart disease.

B. Niacin—most common in corn eaters by deficiency of **tryptophan** that it is used to synthesize niacin. The deficiency causes **pellegra** with skin rashes, decreased posterior column function, spastic lower limbs with weakness, confusion, fatigue, and rigidity.

C. Vitamin B_{12} (cobalamin)

1. Deficiency is usually caused by decreased intrinsic factor production from **pernicious anemia** (autoimmune attack on gastric cells), tumors, infection, parasites, and surgery.

2. Vitamin B_{12} binds **intrinsic factor** (made by the gastric parietal cells) and is absorbed in the **ileum**.

3. Deficiency causes **megaloblastic anemia** (MCV > 100), hypersegmented PMNs, glossitis, anorexia, and diarrhea. **Subacute combined degeneration** of the spinal cord involves the lower cervical and **upper thoracic posterior and lateral columns** and causes **spongiform demyelination**, impaired vibration, proprioception sensation, and paraplegia. The posterior columns are affected first. It may also cause visual deterioration, mental deterioration, and symmetric peripheral neuropathy.

4. Nitrous oxide from inhalation anesthesia inactivates vitamin B_{12} and may increase symptoms.

5. Diagnosis is made by hypersegmented PMNs on a peripheral blood smear, megaloblastic anemia, and vitamin B_{12} assay. The most reliable indication of decreased intracellular cobalamin is **increased serum methylmalonic acid and homocysteine**.

6. Treatment is with B$_{12}$ injections. If treatment is with folic acid, the anemia may be corrected, but the neurologic symptoms may worsen (see Fig. 280).

D. Pyridoxine—deficiency is seen with INH and hydralazine treatment and causes lower limb parasthesias, pain, and weakness.

E. Vitamin A—deficiency causes decreased vision. Increased levels have been associated with **pseudotumor**.

F. Vitamin D—deficiency causes **rickets** with decreased PTH and decreased bone strength.

G. Vitamin E—deficiency is associated with biliary atresia and cystic fibrosis (impaired fat absorption) and causes thick dystrophic axons in the posterior columns with polyneuropathy.

XV. ACQUIRED METABOLIC DISEASES AND BACTERIAL TOXINS

A. **Serum osmolarity = 2(Na + K) + BUN/28 + Glucose/18.**

B. Hypercarbia causes asterixis and papilledema.

C. Hypoglycemia < 30 mg/dL causes symptoms and < 10 mg/dL causes coma.

D. Hepatic encephalopathy

1. It causes **asterixis**, mental status changes, and EEG slow waves. The serum ammonia is usually > 200 mg/dL.

2. **Alzheimer type II** protoplasmic astrocytes form in the deep cortex, basal ganglia, thalamus, SN, cerebellum, and pontine nuclei.

3. The increased **ammonia** that is not converted to urea in the liver may cause increased GABA.

4. Symptoms are worse with constipation, increased protein intake, and GI hemorrhage.

5. Treatment is by decreasing protein intake, injesting lactulose, and neomycin PO to control colon flora.

E. Reye's syndrome—nonicteric hepatic encephalopathy that develops in children with influenza B or varicella and often who have received aspirin. The brain swells and the liver becomes fatty. Mortality is 10%.

F. Uremic encephalopathy—no edema is present. The mechanism is unknown. There is a postdialysis headache by SIADH that lasts for 8 to 48 hours. Uremia also produces a peripheral polyneuropathy.

G. Syndrome of inappropiate ADH (SIADH)—caused by trauma, infection, stroke, medications, and tumors.

H. Hypokalemia—causes muscle weakness and occasionally mental status changes.

I. Hyperkalemia—causes muscle weakness and cardiac arrest.

J. Central pontine myelinolysis (CPM)—there is **no inflammation**. There is decreased myelin in the pons and occasionally in other sites. It is associated with rapid correction of hyponatremia in patients with ETOH abuse, **malnutrition**, renal failure, and burns. Symptoms may include quadriparesis, locked-in syndrome, and pseudobulbar palsy. See Section XI.

K. Hypoparathyroidism—causes hypocalcemia with tetany, cramps, and seizures. Ca^{++} deposits may form in the basal ganglia, dentate nucleus, and cortex cause choreoathetosis, rigidity, and ataxia.

L. Hyperthyroidism—causes tremor.

M. Hypothyroidism causes apathy and neuropathy. If it occurs early in life, it causes **cretinism** with jaundice, mottled skin, wide posterior fontanel, mental retardation, spasticity, and deafness. If it occurs later, it causes **myxedema**.

N. Tetanus

1. Caused by *Clostridium tetani*, and the exotoxin may enter through a cut and moves to the CNS by means of the peripheral nerves.

2. It produces **presynaptic excitation of agonist and antagonist muscles** (especially the masseter causing lockjaw or trismus) by inhibiting the neurotransmitter release of inhibitory neurons (especially **Renshaw cells** in the spinal cord).

3. Local tetanus occurs with wounds on the extremities, causes tightness and spasms, and disappears over a few weeks. Cephalic tetanus occurs with facial wounds. Generalized tetanus is the most common and causes diffuse spasms, trismus, and apnea. It has a 50% mortality.

4. The clinical picture is similar to strychnine poisoning, black widow spider bite, and stiff-man syndrome.

5. The EMG reveals a loss of the silent period after contraction with continuous discharge of normal motor units.

6. Treatment is with antitoxin, penicillin, and wound debridement. Valium, curare, and intubation/tracheostomy may be needed. Active immunization with a booster should be obtained every 10 years.

O. Diphtheria—from *Corynebacterium diphtheriae* and causes throat and tracheal inflammatory exudate with exotoxins that affect the heart and nerves, causing **ascending paralysis** and cardiomyopathy. It is distinguished by early bulbar and ciliary dysfunction and delayed symmetric sensorimotor peripheral neuropathy with demyelination. Treatment is with antitoxin.

P. Botulism—from *Clostridia botulinum*, obtained by contamination in home-canned vegetables or from wound infections. The exotoxin causes **presynaptic inhibition at the NMJ by decreasing ACh** release (similar to Eaton-Lambert syndrome). Symptoms include blurred vision, **unreactive pupils**, diplopia, bulbar paralysis, and then respiratory suppression and quadriparesis in a **descending pattern** that evolves over 2 to 4 days. There are no sensory changes. Diagnose by EMG that may have an incremental response like Eaton-Lambert syndrome. Extraocular muscles recover first. Treatment is with antiserum, guanidine, and supportive respiratory care.

Q. Black widow spider venom—depletes the presynaptic ACh stores into the NMJ, causing cramps and spasms followed by weakness. Treatment is with Ca^{++} gluconate and $MgSO_4$.

XVI. CONGENITAL METABOLIC DISEASES

A. Many of these diseases effect neonates and thus a good neonatal neurologic examination is necessary. Assess for diencephalic function (alertness and responsivity), brain stem and cerebellar function (automatisms such as sucking, rooting, swallowing, and grasping), reticulospinal/cerebellar/spinal function (posture and movements), midbrain and pons function (eye movements), upper brain stem and spinal function with cortical facilitation (Moro/startle and placing reactions), and hypothalamic function (respiration, thirst, and temperature). Monitor food intake to detect failure to thrive.

B. Aminoacidopathies—there are 48 types and they cause mental retardation by 2 years.

   1. Phenylketonuria—the **most frequent type**. Deficiency of phenylalanine hydroxylase in the liver that is needed to convert phenylalanine to tyrosine. Phenylalanine accumulates and causes defective myelination. Inheritance is autosomal recessive on chromosome 12. Diagnose by increased urine phenylpyruvic acid and serum phenylalanine. Typically it affects fair-skinned children with blue eyes and causes a musty odor. Treatment is by limiting intake of L-phenylalanine to decrease mental retardation.

   2. Homocysteinuria—causes a defect in **methionine** metabolism. There is decreased collagen and elastin in vessels. There is increased homocysteine in the blood, urine, and CSF. Inheritance is autosomal recessive. It is physically similar to Marfan's syndrome (tall and thin) but with **mental retardation** and increased incidence of **strokes**, lens dislocations, and arachnodactyly.

   3. Maple syrup urine disease—causes decreased **branched-chain amino acid** catabolism. Inheritance is autosomal recessive. Death occurs by 4 weeks unless leucine, isoleucine, and valine intake is limited.

C. Sphingolipidoses—lysosomal storage diseases caused by enzyme deficiency with accumulation in the lysosomes of various products from glycolytic or peptide degradation. There is accumulation of lipids including cholesterol, cerebrosides, and phospholipids. Sphingomyelin is a phospholipid with sphingosine. Ceramide is sphingosine with a long chain fatty acid. Sphingomyelin is ceramide and phosphocholine. Cerebroside is ceramide and a hexose. Ganglioside is ceramide and sialic acid. Gray matter has more gangliosides and less phopholipids than white matter. White matter is 60% lipid, whereas gray matter is 35%. Accumulation of these products damages neurons and myelin sheaths.

   1. Neimann-Pick disease—caused by a deficiency of **sphingomyelinase** with accumulation of sphingomyelin and cholesterol. Inheritance autosomal recessive. It occurs usually in infants 3 to 9 months with death in 2 years. There is a predilection for Ashkenasi Jews. It causes cherry-red maculae (50%), supranuclear paresis of vertical gaze, psychomotor retardation, hepatosplenomegaly, and normal head size; Neimann-Pick cells or **"foam cells"** are large vacuolated histiocytes and lymphocytes. Accumulation occurs in the brain stem, cerebellum, spinal cord, and visceral organs.

2. Gaucher's disease—the most frequent sphingolipidosis. There is a deficiency of **glucocerebrosidase** with accumulation of glucocerebrosides. Inheritance is autosomal recessive. It usually develops in late childhood and is usually nonneuropathic with accumulation in the liver, spleen, marrow, and lung with symptomatic hypersplenism with anemia and thrombocytopenia. There are rare infantile and juvenile forms affecting neurons and causing death by 2 years. There is a predilection for Ashkenasi Jews. **Gaucher cells** have wrinkled tissue paper appearance from stored glucocerebroside.

3. Fabry's disease—caused by a deficiency of **α-galactosidase** with accumulation of **ceramides**. Inheritance is **X-linked** recessive with onset in adolescence. It causes **pain episodes** and dysesthesias. Deposits accumulate in blood vessel walls, cornea, kidneys, cardiac muscle fibers, and noncortical neurons. Symptons include hypertension, renal failure, congestive heart failure, and death by myocardial infarction or stroke usually in the **sixth decade**.

4. Tay-Sachs disease—caused by a deficiency of **hexosaminidase A** with accumulation of **GM$_2$ gangliosides**. Inheritance is autosomal recessive with onset by 6 months and death by 4 years. There is a predilection for Ashkenasi Jews. It causes **cherry-red maculae** by retinal ganglion cell degeneration allowing vascular choroid to be visible and **macrocephaly** without visceromegaly. Accumulation occurs in the gray matter.

5. Sandhoff's disease—caused by a deficiency of **hexosaminidase A and B** with accumulation of **GM$_2$ gangliosides**. There is no predilection for Jews. It has a similar clinical picture to Tay-Sachs disease but has visceral storage in the liver, spleen, kidney, and heart.

6. GM$_1$ gangliosidosis—caused by a deficiency of acid β-galactosidase with accumulation of GM$_1$ gangliosides. Inheritance is autosomal recessive with onset in 3 months and death in 2 years. There is both CNS and visceral involvement with dysmorphic face, cherry-red maculae, hepatosplenomegaly, bone abnormalities, and contractures.

D. Mucopolysaccharidoses—enzyme deficiencies of mucopolysaccharide degradation producing lipid accumulation in the lysosomes of the gray matter (causing neuronal death) and polysaccharide accumulation in the connective tissue.

1. Hurler's disease (MPS1H)—caused by a deficiency of **α-L-iduronidase** with accumulation of mucopolysaccharides (MPS). The urine contains **heparin and dermatan sulfate**. Inheritance is autosomal recessive with onset at 1 year and death by 5 to 10 years from cardiac or respiratory causes. Symptoms include **gargoyle face**, **mental retardation**, **corneal opacities**, conduction deafness, hepatosplenomegaly, cardiac dysfunction, skeletal abnormalities, and thick meninges that may cause spinal cord compression. Neurons are enlarged (**Figs. 186 and 187**).

2. Scheie's syndrome (MPS1S or 5) is a milder rare form of Hurler's disease with autosomal recessive inheritance. **There is no mental retardation** or neuronal storage. It may produce spinal cord compression from thickened dura, corneal opacities, and carpal tunnel syndrome.

3. Hunter's syndrome (MPS2)—caused by a deficiency of **iduronate sulfatase**. The urine contains **heparin and dermatan sulfate**. Inheritance is **X-linked** recessive. Presentation is similar to Hurler's disease but milder with **no mental retardation**, less corneal clouding and slower

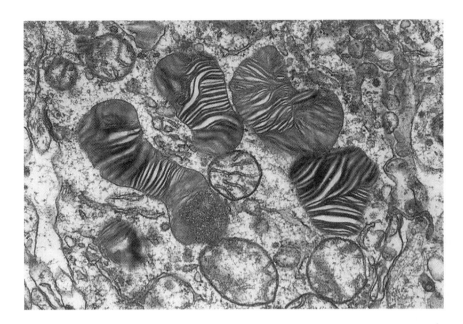

Figure 186   Hurler's disease (electron micrograph). "Zebra bodies" of stored gangliosides. (From Schochet SS Jr. Intoxications and disease of the central nervous system. In: Nelson JS, Parisi JE, Schochet SS Jr (Eds.). Principles and Practice of Neuropathology. St. Louis, MO: Mosby, 1993:334. With permission.)

progression. There is characteristic **skin pebbling** and peripheral nerve entrapments. Patients may survive to adulthood.

4. Sanfilippo's syndrome (MPS3)—caused by deficiencies of multiple enzymes. The urine contains **heparin sulfate**. Inheritance is autosomal recessive. It produces mental retardation and neurologic symptoms but less corneal clouding and skeletal abnormalities.

5. Morquio's syndrome (MPS4)—caused by a deficiency of galactose 6-sulfatase and β-galactosidase. The urine contains **keratan sulfate**. Inheritance is autosomal recessive. There is **no mental retardation** but severe skeletal deformities with **ligamentous laxities and odontoid hypoplasia and thick cervical dura** with cervical myelopathy, dwarfism, and osteoporosis.

6. Maroteaux-Lamy disease (MPS6)—caused by a deficiency of arylsulfatase B. The urine contains **dermatan sulfate**. Inheritance is autosomal recessive. There is no mental retardation but there may be compressive myelopathy and hepatosplenomegaly.

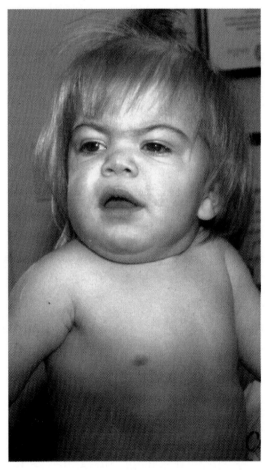

Figure 187   Hurler's disease. "Gargoyle face." (From Matalon RK. Disorders of mucopolysaccharide metabolism. In: Nelson WE (Senior Editor), Behrman RE, Kliegman RM, Arvin AM (Eds.). Nelson Textbook of Pediatrics, 15th ed. Philadelphia, PA: W.B. Saunders, 1996:398. With permission.)

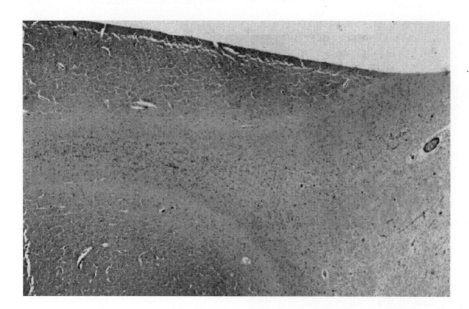

Figure 188   Metachromatic leukodystrophy (H and E). Demyelination with U-fiber sparing.

7. Sly's syndrome (MPS7)—caused by a deficiency of β-glucuronidase. The urine contains **dermatan sulfate, heparin sulfate, and chondroitin sulfate**. Inheritance is autosomal recessive. There is moderate mental retardation, corneal clouding, hepatosplenomegaly, and bony changes.

E. Leukodystrophies—caused by enzyme deficiencies with abnormal formation, destruction, or maintenance of myelin. They mainly affect white matter.

1. Krabbe's disease (globoid cell leukodystrophy)—caused by a deficiency of **galactocerebroside β-galactosidase** with accumulation of galactocerebroside from myelin sheaths in lysosomes. Inheritance is autosomal recessive with onset 3 to 6 months and death by 2 years. It causes psychomotor delay and microcephaly. There is cavitation of the white matter, with **sparing of the subcortical U-fibers**. The basal ganglia and thalamus appear hyperdense on CT. **Globoid cells** are large macrophages around blood vessels. **Psychosine** accumulation kills oligodendrocytes.

2. Metachromatic leukodystrophy—the **most common leukodystrophy**. There is a deficiency of **arylsulfatase A** with **accumulation of sulfatides** in lysosomes. Inheritance is autosomal recessive on chromosome 22 with usually late infantile onset at 1 to 4 years with death in 3 years. It causes psychomotor deterioration. There is cavitation of the white matter with **sparing of the subcortical U-fibers** and degeneration of PNS myelin. It also damages the liver, spleen, and kidneys. The Hirsh-Peiffer reaction is with acidic cresyl-violet aniline dye causing cells with sulfatides to change to a brown color instead of purple. (**Fig. 188**).

3. Adrenoleukodystrophy (ALD)—caused by a deficiency of **lipid oxidation in peroxisomes** with accumulation of **long chain fatty acids**. Inheritance is **X-linked** recessive so it affects males. Onset is 3 to 10 years with death in 3 to 5 years. Symptoms start with behavioral and intellectual deterioration followed by visual, auditory, and motor decline and **adrenal insufficiency with bronze skin**. There is cavitation of the **parieto-occipital white matter**.

4. Pelizaeus-Merzbacher disease—caused by defective synthesis of proteolipid apoprotein, a myelin basic protein (MBP) that is required for oligodendrocyte differentiation and survival. Inheritance is **X-linked** recessive so it usually affects males. Onset is in infancy with death in young adulthood. It produces an atrophic brain with demyelination that spares perivascular

white matter. There is a **tigroid pattern** on MRI from intact and degenerating myelin. Symptoms include abnormal eye movements, spasticity, ataxia, and mental retardation. It is the **only leukodystrophy with 100% incidence of nystagmus**.

5. Canavan's disease—caused by a deficiency of **N-acetyl-aspartoacylase**. There is increased urine *N*-acetylaspartic acid. Inheritance is autosomal recessive with a predilection for Ashkenasi Jews. Onset is in infancy with death by 5 years. There is **spongy white matter degeneration** with vacuoles that **preferentially affects subcortical U-fibers**. The **brain actually increases in size**; psychomotor regression, blindness, and spasticity.

6. Alexander's disease—the deficiency is unknown and there is sporadic inheritance with no clear genetic transmission. Onset is in infancy with death by 3 years. There is hemispheric demyelination with **macrocephaly** and mitochondrial dysfunction. It mainly affects the **frontal lobe** with white matter demyelination. **Rosenthal fibers** (eosinophylic hyalin bodies that are likely glial degeneration products) form especially periventricular, perivascular, and subpial. Symptoms include psychomotor retardation and seizures.

7. Sudanophyllic leukodystrophy—onset at 3 months with death in 2 years or there may be delayed onset 3 to 7 years with a chronic course. There is a diffuse degeneration of medullated fibers with phagocytosis of sudanophillic myelin products. Symptoms include spasticity, blindness, and psychomotor regression.

F. Other metabolic disorders

1. Menke's kinky hair disease—caused by a **defect in copper absorption in the GI tract** (opposite of Wilson's disease). Inheritance is **X-linked recessive** with death before 2 years. There is diffuse loss of all neurons, tortuous vessels, and metaphyseal spurring. Secondary hair growth is **brittle**, twisted, and colorless. Symptoms include seizures and **mental retardation**.

2. Leigh's disease (subacute necrotic encephalomyelopathy)—**mitochondrial dysfunction** by multiple metabolic defects. There may be a deficiency of cytochrome C oxidase. Inheritance is autosomal recessive with onset before 1 year. There is **bilateral symmetric spongiform degeneration** and necrosis of the thalamus, **basal ganglia**, brain stem, and spinal cord with peripheral nerve demyelination. Symptoms include decreased muscle tone and head control, seizures, myoclonus, ophthalmoplegia, and respiratory and swallowing problems.

3. Lowe syndrome (oculo-cerebro-renal syndrome)—an X-linked recessive disease causing bilateral cataracts, large eyes, nystagmus, psychomotor retardation, and death by renal failure.

4. Ataxia-telangiectasia—caused by **defective DNA repair** with autosomal recessive inheritance. Death occurs by 20 years from infection or lymphoma. There is degeneration of CNS and decreased antibodies.

5. Lesch-Nyhan disease—X-linked recessive inheritance with deficiency of HGPRT enzyme. There is accumulation of uric acid with self-mutilation and choreoathetosis.

6. Zellweger syndrome (cerebro-hepato-renal syndrome)—autosomal recessive inheritance with death in a few months. There are decreased liver peroxisomes and accumulation of long-chain fatty acids. There is cortical dysgenesis and white matter degeneration with hepatorenal dysfunction.

XVII. DEGENERATIVE DISEASES

A. They usually occur in older patients. The CSF protein is usually slightly elevated but with a normal cell count. Atrophy is slow deterioration accompanied by little gliosis, whereas degenerative diseases have a more rapid progression and more gliosis. A slow deterioration over many years may appear to have a sudden onset when a system's neuronal loss exceeds its "safety factor." Degenerative diseases are usually bilaterally symmetric with certain systems involved as a result of selective vulnerability (i.e., Purkinje's cells to hyperthermia, cerebellar granular layer to mercury, and hippocampus to hypoxia).

B. Alzheimer's disease

1. It is the most frequent cause of dementia (66%). Onset is after 45 years, usually around 80 years, and it affects 7% of the population after 65 years. There is no sex predilection. Inheritance is usually sporadic but is occasionally dominant with multiple chromosomal associations. Risk is increased with family history, age, less education, trauma, myocardial infarction, and **Down syndrome**.

2. There is **diffuse atrophy** with decreased neurons and synapses in the neocortex and hippocampus. There are **neurofibrillary tangles** (intracytoplasmic, paired helical filaments, immunoreactive for **tau protein**, stain with silver, most frequent in hippocampus and adjacent temporal lobe) and **neuritic plaques** (intracytoplasmic of multiple processes, paired helical filaments, core of β/α^4 **protein amyloid**, stain with silver). These both occur normally with aging but are increased in Alzheimer's disease. There are **Hirano bodies** (rod-shaped eosin inclusions); **decreased neurotransmitters (especially ACh with decreased neurons in the nucleus basalis of Meynert)** and granulovacuolar degeneration of neurons (especially in the hippocampus) (**Fig. 189**).

3. Symptoms start with forgetfulness and then lead to confusion, ideomotor apraxia, dysnomia, and akinetic mutism. There are usually no major cortical deficits such as hemiplegia, sensory loss, or visual deterioration. The temporoparietal area is usually affected first.

4. Diagnosis is made by history, examination, CT or MRI (that demonstrates atrophy and enlarged ventricles), and by ruling out treatable causes of dementia.

5. There is no treatment.

C. Pick's disease—onset 40 to 60 years with female predominance. Inheritance is sporadic but occasionally dominant. Symptoms are similar to Alzheimer's disease but with increased frontal lobe dysfunction (impaired social restraint, etc.). There is **frontotemporal atrophy** without pathologic changes of Alzheimer's disease. It spares the superior posterior temporal gyrus. **Pick bodies** (intracytoplasmic eosinophilic inclusions) form especially in the hippocampus. It affects gray and white matter. Death occurs in 2 to 5 years.

D. Huntington's disease—onset in the 30s, with survival 15 to 30 years more. There are 10 cases in 100,000 people. Inheritance is autosomal **dominant** on **chromosome 4** with no sex predilection. Symptoms begin with personality changes (suspicious, etc.) followed by subcortical dementia (no aphasia, agnosia, or apraxia) and choreoform movements (affects hands and face first). There is **atrophy mostly of the caudate** (with boxcar ventricles) more than the putamen, GP, and cortex. Medium spiny type 1 neu-

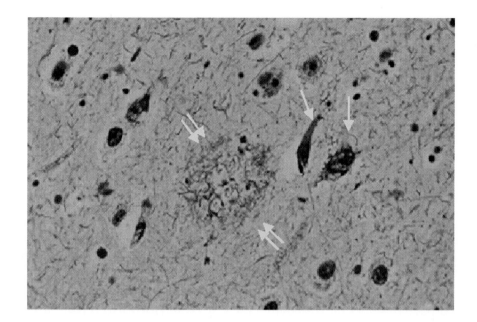

Figure 189 Alzheimer's disease (silver). A neuritic plaque (double arrows) and neurofibrillary tangles (single arrows).

rons are affected first and aspiny neurons are spared. There is **decreased GABA and ACh** and increased NE and somatostatin. Haloperidal (Haldol) 2 to 10 mg/day may be used to treat the athetosis, with low doses and frequent drug holidays to decrease the risk of tardive dyskinesia (**Fig. 190**).

E. Wilson's disease (hepatolenticular degeneration)—autosomal recessive inheritance on chromosome 13 with male predominance. There is **accumulation of copper** in the brain **with decreased ceruloplasmin and serum copper**, and **increased urine copper**. The CT has **hypodense** basal ganglia. **Kayser-Fleis-**

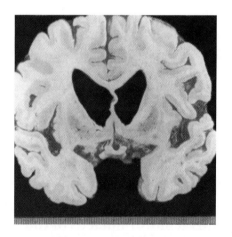

Figure 190 Huntington's disease. Gross specimen with atrophic caudates and "box-car" ventricles.

cher gold rings form in the deepest corneal layer around the iris. There is neurologic and psychologic deterioration with tremor, dysarthria, and rigidity; spongy red degeneration and cavitation of the **putamen and GP** with occasional atrophy of the superior and middle frontal gyri. **Alzheimer II** astrocytes with large vesicular nuclei form in the gray matter of the cerebrum, cerebellum, and brain stem. **Opalski cells** form in the GP. Onset is 10 to 30 years and liver disease starts before 20 years and leads to cirrhosis and splenomegaly. Treat by limiting foods high in copper (i.e., liver and chocolate) and chelate copper with D-**penicillamine**. With treatment there may be disappearance of KF rings and improvement of liver function tests.

F. Fahr's disease (idiopathic basal ganglia calcification)—primary basal ganglia and cerebellar blood vessel calcification associated with renal disease or decreased parathyroid hormone. It may also involve the dentate nuclei.

G. Progressive supranuclear palsy (Steele-Richardson-Olzewski syndrome)—onset of 50 to 60 years and death within 1 to 12 years with male predominance. It occasionally occurs after a bout with pneumonia. Symptoms include deterioration of intellect, vision, speech, and **gait**, with **vertical gaze palsy**, loss of voluntary eye movements and opticokinetic nystagmus, decreased oculocephalic reflexes, **pseudobulbar palsy**, and axial rigidity without tremor. There is **atrophy of the midbrain**, superior colliculus, and subthalmic nuclei with ventricular dilation and decreased neurons in the GP, SN, and various brain stem nuclei. The neurofibrillary tangles are different than Alzheimer-type. "Bulb" is an old term for the medulla.

H. Striatonigral degeneration—onset around 50 years. Symptoms include rigidity and akinesia (Parkinson-like symptoms) with syncope. There are atrophic and brown **putamen** and depigmented **SN** as well as decreased neurons in the putamen, caudate, and SN. There are **no Lewy bodies** or neurofibrillary tangles.

I. Hallervorden-Spatz disease—onset in late childhood with death in early adulthood. The disease is progressive over 20 years. It usually has sporadic onset with occasional recessive inheritence. Symptoms include extrapyramidal and corticospinal dysfunction with dementia. CT has **hypodense basal ganglia**. There are brown atrophic GP and SN secondary to **iron deposition**.

J. Acquired hepatocerebral degeneration—occurs with chronic liver disease and is increased with elevated ammonia levels. It is associated with long-term TPN (by manganese toxicity). T1-weighted MRI shows hyperintense basal ganglia. There is pseudolaminar necrosis with gray/white junction changes.

K. Parkinson's disease (paralysis agitans)

1. Onset is 40 to 50 years with male predominance. It affects 1% of the population older than 50 years and there are 200 cases in 100,000 people.

2. **Bradykinesia** (slow to initiate and execute movements), **resting pill-rolling tremor**, **rigidity**, abnormal gait, and dementia (10 to 15%).

3. Pathology—**decreased neuromelanin and neurons in the SNpc, locus ceruleus, and dorsal motor nucleus of the vagus**. There are neuronal intracytoplasmic **Lewy bodies** (from neurofilaments, laminated, eosinophilic core, clear halo, occasionally in other diseases or in normal people) and decreased DA in the caudate and putamen. It may be idiopathic or secondary to encephalitis (after von Economo's viral encephalitis in 1930 with no Lewy bodies), manganese, carbon monoxide, and MPTP toxicity. Parkinson-plus is multisystem atrophy (**Fig. 191**).

4. Diffuse Lewy body disease—occurs in cortical neurons and may be a variant.

5. The rate-limiting enzyme in DA production is tyrosine β-hydroxylase.

6. Treatment—(a) **carbidopa (Sinemet)** (L-DOPA and carbidopa, a decarboxylase inhibitor), (b) **amantadine** (increases dopamine release, anticholinergic), (c) **benztropine (Cogentin) or** trihexylphenidyl (**Artane**) (anticholinergics, may cause slow mentation and cause constipation), (d) **bromocriptine or pergolide** (stimulates D2 receptors), and (e) selegiline (**Eldepryl**) (MAO-b inhibitor, decreases degradation of DA, and slows disease progression). Try to limit protein intake because amino acids antagonize L-DOPA; initial therapy is with selegiline amantadine, benztropine, or propranolol (for tremor); therapy for more severe disease is with Sinemet.

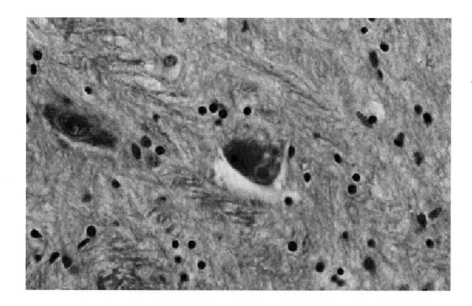

Figure 191   Parkinson's disease (H and E). Lewy bodies (neuronal intracytoplasmic inclusion with an eosinophilic core surrounded by a clear halo).

7. Surgical options—lesioning of the contralateral VL thalamus or GPi (best for tremor or rigidity, less effective for akinesia) stimulation of these structures and the subthalamus, and implantation of adrenal medulla or fetal SN tissue. Previous treatment included ligation of the **anterior choroidal artery.** Survival is 80% at 10 years with two-thirds disabled in 5 years.

L. Multisystem atrophy—25% of patients with Parkinson's symptoms have poor response to DA. Consider Parkinson-plus syndrome with multisystem atrophy including Shy-Drager syndrome, striatonigral degeneration, progressive supranuclear palsy, and olivopontocerebellar degeneration with autonomic dysfunction (decreased sweating, impotence, incontinence, and orthostatic hypotension).

1. Shy-Drager syndrome—onset at 50 to 60 years and death within 7 years. There is no sex predilection and inheritance is sporadic. There are Parkinson's symptoms without Lewy bodies and with **autonomic dysfunction.** There is loss of cells in the intermediolateral column of the spinal cord and putamen.

2. Olivopontocerebellar atrophy—onset at 15 years with sporadic, recessive, and dominant inheritance. **Ataxia of the lower limbs** occurs first. There is atrophy of the pons, **middle cerebellar peduncle,** inferior olive, and cerebellar cortex. It is associated with Parkinson's syndrome.

M. Diffuse Lewy body disease—dementia with increased frontal atrophy, parkinsonian features, and eosinophilic **intracytoplasmic** inclusions.

N. Friedreich's ataxia—the **most frequent hereditary ataxia.** Onset is before 20 years with death in mid-30s and inability to walk 5 years after onset. There is autosomal recessive inheritance on **chromosome 9** and no sex predilection. It is associated with cardiomyopathy and diabetes. There is degeneration of axons and myelin in the **posterior columns and corticospinal tracts,** more prominent distally. It also affects the **spinocerebellar tracts,** cerebellum (decreased Purkinje's cells in the superior vermis), inferior olive, brain stem nuclei (CNs VIII, X, and XII), and DRG. It **spares motor neurons** and mainly affects large peripheral myelinated fibers. Symptoms begin with gait ataxia followed by upper limb and speech disturbances. Mental status remains normal.

O. Familial myoclonic epilepsy

1. Lafora's body disease—onset in the mid-teens and autosomal recessive inheritance. Symptoms include myoclonic seizures and dementia. There is brain atrophy and diffuse neuronal Lafora's bodies (round basophillic polyglucosans) also found in the heart, muscle, and liver.

2. Baltic myoclonus—onset before 11 years and autosomal recessive inheritance. There are myoclonic seizures and Purkinje's cell atrophy.

P. Motor neuron disease

1. Spinal muscular atrophy—degeneration of the anterior horn and hypoglossal nuclei with sparing of the corticospinal tracts and bulbar nuclei.

   (a) Werdnig-Hoffman disease (SMA type 1, infantile)—onset from 0 to 6 months and death within 1.5 years from pneumonia. It is the **most common spinal muscle atrophy**. It has autosomal **recessive** inheritance on **chromosome 5q**. Atrophy is most severe in the proximal extensors and trunk. The extraocular muscles are spared; no mental retardation.

   (b) Wohlfart-Kugelberg-Welander disease (SMA type 2)—onset usually before 5 years (although it may be up to 17 years) with death usually by 5 to 10 years. There is male predominance and different forms have autosomal recessive, dominant, and X-linked inheritance (on chromosome 5). Symptoms are bilateral and symmetric with proximal limbs affected first.

   (c) SMA type 3—adult onset with multiple forms with sporadic, **dominant**, recessive, and X-linked inheritance. It is slowly progressive.

2. Amyotrophic lateral sclerosis—the most frequent adult-onset progressive motor neuron disease. Onset is around 55 years with death 50% in 3 years and 90% in 6 years. There is a slight male predominance with sporadic inheritance but 10% are dominant on chromosome 21. There is **degeneration of motor neurons (including Betz's cells) and the corticospinal tracts**. Ther are **UMN and LMN signs** with **fasciculations in all extremities** and **diffuse hyperreflexia**. Symptoms usually begin in the hands and there is progressive bulbar palsy with face and tongue weakness. Bladder control is maintained. There are no sensory changes. **Bunina bodies** (intracytoplasmic, anterior horn cells) form. Amyotrophy is denervation atrophy of muscle. There may be antibodies to gangliosides. EMG demonstrates fasciculations and fibrillations (see Fig. 276).

Q. Memory aid

1. X-linked metabolic diseases—Fabry's, Hunter's, adrenoleukodystrophy, Pelezius-Merzbacher, Menke's kinky hair, Lowe's, and Lesch-Nyhan. Most others are recessive with a few indeterminate.

2. Autosomal dominant diseases—Wohlfart-Kugelberg-Welander disease and Huntington's chorea.

3. Adolescent regression of intellect and behavioral changes—Wilson's, Hallervorden-Spatz, Lafora's body, Gaucher's, mucopolysaccharidosis, metachromatic leukodystrophy, and GM_2 gangliosidosis.

4. Metabolic diseases that may have adult onset—Metachromatic adrenoleukodystrophy, adrenoleukodystrophy, Krabbe's disease, GM_2 gangliosidosis, Wilson's disease, Leigh's disease, Neimann-Pick disease, Gaucher's disease, mucopolysaccharidoses, Refsum's disease, and porphyria.

5. Strokes in children—Fabry's disease, homocysteinuria.

6. Parkinson's symptoms in adolescents—Wilson's disease, Hallervorden-Spatz disease.

7. Cerebellar degeneration—Ethanol, phenytoin (Dilantin), paraneoplastic syndrome, Down syndrome, and Freidriech's ataxia.

8. Mitochondrial DNA diseases—**Kearns-Sayre syndrome** (autosomal dominant transmission, elevated serum pyruvate, and associated with retinitis pigmentosum), Leber's hereditary optic atrophy, Leigh's subacute necrotizing encephalopathy, Luft's disease, MELAS, and MERRF.

XVIII. DEMYELINATING DISEASES

A. Myelin

1. CNS myelin–associated proteins are myelin basic protein (MBP) and proteolipid protein. PNS myelin—associated proteins are MBP, P2, and Po.

2. The CNS and PNS myelin have different protein and lipid components and different periodicity of lamellae. The CNS myelin does not regenerate well.

3. Primary demyelination is by processes that affect myelin or myelin-forming cells. Segmental demyelination is myelin loss with preserved axons.

B. Peripheral demyelination

1. Toxic—Diphtheria (toxin inhibits Schwann cell myelin synthesis mainly in the DRG and ventral and dorsal roots, where the blood-nerve barrier is leaky, and causes segmental demyelination), lead, and hexachlorophene.

2. Immune mediated

(a) **Guillain-Barré** (idiopathic polyneuritis)—rapid onset, and occurs with trauma, surgery, infection, immunization, and neoplasm. It is usually **monophasic** but occasionally relapsing. It involves the DRG, ventral and dorsal nerve roots, and **peripheral nerves**. It affects mainly **motor and autonomic function**. There are perivascular mononuclear infiltrates and segmental demyelination. The CSF reveals normal pressure, **acellularity** (90%), and increased protein after 5 weeks. Treatment is with **plasmapheresis**. Steroids have not been shown to help.

(b) Experimental allergic neuritis—caused by T-cell attack of the P2 protein by cell-mediated immunity.

3. Metabolic—diabetes mellitus, uremia, and hypothyroidism.

C. Hypertrophic (onion bulb) neuropathies—caused by repeated demyelination-remyelinations and seen with Dejerine-Sottas, Charcot-Marie-Tooth, and Refsum's diseases. Schwann cell processes and collagen layers surround the axons and myelin.

D. Central demyelination

    1. Immune-mediated

        (a) Multiple sclerosis (**MS**)

            (i) Peak age 20 to 40 years, with female predominance. The highest incidence is in Northern Europe. The **risk** is related to one's geographic location before age 15 years. Influences are considered to be latitude (distance from the equator), familial (15% have an affected relative), infectious, and autoimmune. The findings are visual (**optic neuritis** 25%, most improve in 2 weeks, and one-third recover completely), autonomic, and sensorimotor (50%).

            (ii) Lhermitte's sign is common. Charcot's triad is nystagmus, **scanning speech**, and intention tremor. **Bilateral** internuclear ophthalmoplegia (**INO**) is almost pathognomonic. Trigeminal neuralgia and bladder spasticity also occur. Fifty percent of patients that have optic neuritis will get MS.

            (iii) It is usually **relapsing/remitting** (Charcot type) and 10% of cases are progressive. Relapse rate is 0.4 attacks per year with 30% occurring in the first year and 50% in the second year. The 25-year survival is 74% compared with 86% of the rest of the population in a study from Rochester, Minnesota. Pregnancy does not increase the relapse rate. Diagnosis is made by MRI (85% sensitive), CSF oligoclonal bands, and visual evoked potentials (abnormal in 80%, BAER and SSEP may also be abnormal) (**Fig. 192**).

            (iv) CSF has increased protein but seldom >100 mg/dL, increased macrophages, **IgG index** (CSF/serum IgG $\div$ CSF/serum albumin) is >1.7, and **oligoclonal bands** (also seen with SSPE and syphilis). There may be increased CSF MBP during an exacerbation. Gross pathologic examination reveals plaques (acute are pink and older are gray) that are gelatinous, firm, ovoid, **perpendicular to the ventricles**, and in the superolateral **periventricular white matter** (where the subependymal veins line the ventricles), corpus callosum, subcortical white matter, optic nerves/chiasm/and tracts (90%), brain stem, and spinal cord (especially subpial where veins are near white matter).

            (v) **Dawson's fingers** are perivenular extensions of inflammation into the deep white matter. **The plaques do not extend past the root entry zone (REZ) into the peripheral nerves.** The posterior fossa is more commonly affected in children. Microscopic examination of an active plaque demonstrates decreased myelin, macrophages, destruction or proliferation of oligodendrocytes, **axonal sparing**, perivascular lymphocytes (T $>$ B cells), parenchymal T4 cells, perivascular T8 cells and B cells, reactive astrocytosis, and edema (**Fig. 193**).

            (vi) Remyelination may occur at the periphery. Inactive plaques have few cells, sharp margins, no oligodendrocytes, and naked axons and astrocytes. MS is similar to

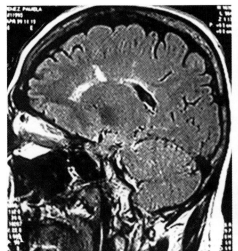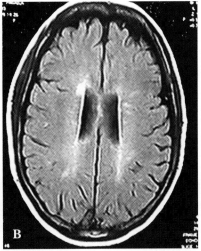

Figure 192   MS. Sagittal (A) and axial (B) infused T1-weighted MRIs demonstrate periventricular white matter enhancement with perivenular extension (Dawson's finger).

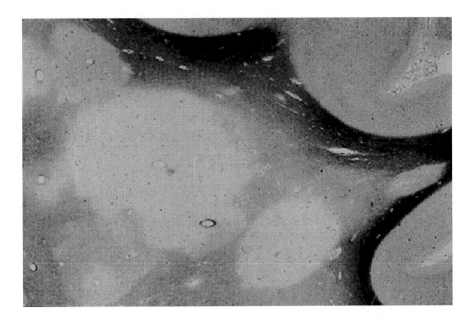

Figure 193   MS (LFB). Multiple white matter demyelinated plaques.

EAM and is transferable by **T cells**. MS may be caused by a postviral autoimmune reaction to MBP or antibodies to oligodendrocytes. Decreased Ts/Th ratio is associated with flareups.

(vii) Treatment is with ACTH, steroids (help to decrease attack duration but not with optic neuritis), and **β-interferon** (decreases attack rate). δ-interferon increases attack rate. Future treatment may involve a copolymer of MBP.

(viii) Acute MS—monophasic, diffuse, larger plaques, may be rapidly fatal, and is more common in Japan.

(ix) Neuromyelitis optica (**Devic's disease**)—a variant of acute MS in adults, primarily affects optic nerves (unilateral or bilateral optic neuritis with blindness) and spinal cord (acute necrotizing transverse myelitis), often rapidly progressive, occasionally fatal, and is more common in Japan.

(x)   Balo's concentric sclerosis—acute MS in young adults, fatal, and has a concentric loss of myelin.

(xi) **Schilder's disease**—affects children, not familial like the leukodystrophies, **aggressive** bilateral acute MS-type demyelination, **hemispheric involvement**, may also affect axons, and is usually fatal.

(b) Acute disseminated encephalomyelitis—postinfectious, monophasic, occurs after a viral illness or vaccination (smallpox or rabies), occasionally fatal but most recover. There is perivenous demyelination with axonal sparing and mononuclear infiltration. It is an autoimmune response to a CNS antigen possibly from the virus and is likely a T-cell response to MBP like EAM.

(c) Acute hemorrhagic leukoencephalitis (Weston-Hurst disease)—monophasic, rapid progression, fatal, occurs after a respiratory infection, drugs, or immunizations, and causes white matter edema and hemorrhages.

(d) Experimental allergic encephalomyelitis (EAM)—an experimental MS model, caused by a T cell–mediated immune response to MBP.

2.   Infectious—PML, SSPE, rubella (like SSPE but without intranuclear inclusions), and HIV.

3.   Ischemic—Binswanger's encephalopathy, carbon monoxide (may initially survive and then develop symptoms days later due to white matter degeneration), and chronic edema (spares subcortical U-fibers).

4.   Metabolic demyelination (leukodystrophy)—widespread confluent myelin loss, astrocytosis, minimal inflammation (except adrenoleukodystrophy with perivascular lymphocytes), and sparing of subcortical U-fibers (except Canavan's disease).

5.   Iatrogenic—central pontine myelinolysis.

XIX. ISCHEMIA AND HYPOXIA

A. The brain receives 15% of the cardiac output, uses 20% of the blood's O_2, and uses 15% of the blood's glucose. Effects of ischemia depend on the level of flow, duration, collateral flow, location, temperature, age, and serum glucose level (increased lactate formation by the glia causes acidosis that may worsen ischemic damage). The ischemic neurons accumulate Ca^{++}, Na^+, Cl^-, and water. Anaerobic glycolysis causes acidosis and increased extracellular glutamate and free radicals.

B. Early changes at the cellular level

1.   6 hours—neuronal changes and edema, microvacuolation (by dilated mitochondria), shrunken hyperchromatic cells, shrunken cells with incrustations on the surface and cytoplasmic bulging, and homogenous cell changes seen at 6 to 12 hours after injury. These changes may

be due to decreased energy or the abnormal release of excitatory neurotranmitters causing a metabolic cascade.

2. 24 hours—PMNs accumulate.

3. 48 hours—PMN concentration peaks.

4. 3 to 5 days—some macrophages arrive.

5. 2 weeks—vessels start to form around the periphery and enhancement begins.

C. The astrocytes swell and accumulate glycogen and filaments. The oligodendrocytes swell and the microglia form rod cells and ingest debris. All the mechanisms of cell death are associated with increased intracellular Ca^{++}. Delayed neuronal death (maturation phenomenon) is caused by reperfusion with altered ionic homeostasis, lactate accumulation, increased excitatory neurotransmitters, free radicals, and prostaglandins (causing vasoconstriction).

D. **Ischemic penumbra**—the zone of isoelectric silence where the CBF is 8 to 23 mL/100 g/min. The low blood flow prevents neuronal depolarization but does not yet cause ionic changes leading to cell death. The neurons do not function but are still salvageable. Normal CBF is 50 to 55 mL/100 g/min. At a level less than 8, there is ionic pump failure and rapid cell death. The blood vessels in the brain respond to decreased flow first by vasodilating to increase the CBF and then by increasing the O_2 extraction. They are unable to compensate when the CBF is < 20.

CBF (mL/100 g/min)	0	10	15	18
Time until death (min)	< 4	40	80	Infinite

E. Selective vulnerability—all neurons have different vulnerabilities to ischemia that may be related to local changes in vascular supply or cellular differences such as differences in zinc or LDH concentrations. The most vulnerable cells are in the hippocampus, cortex (parieto-occipital deep sulci **third, fifth, and sixth layers**), basal ganglia (**caudate and putamen**), and cerebellum (**Purkinje's cells**). In the hippocampus, the **CA1 (Sommer's area) and CA3 (end plate)** areas are most susceptible and the CA2 area is the resistant sector. The white matter **U-fibers**, the extreme and external capsules, and the claustrum are fairly resistant because they receive dual blood supplies. With ischemia, premature babies have periventricular leukomalacia with spastic diplegia because the germinal matrix is in a watershed zone. In full-term babies, there is loss of cortex and subcortical white matter. In children and adults, there is loss of the deep gray structures, hippocampus, brain stem, and cerebellum. The watershed areas are between the ACA/MCA and MCA/PCA distributions.

F. Hypoxic-ischemic encephalopathy—due to global hypoperfusion or hypoxia. Symptoms are the **"man in a barrel" syndrome** with weakness mainly in the proximal upper limbs, and the stroke usually forms at the border zones in the parieto-occipital area (at the junction of the ACA and MCA/PCA). There may also be **laminar necrosis** of cortical layers 3, 5, and 6 and the putamen.

G. Symptoms of global ischemia range from light-headedness and syncope to coma and death. Hippocampal damage may result in long-term memory deficits.

H. Excitatory neurotransmitters—glutamate and aspartate. The NMDA receptor binds glutamate, causes an influx of Ca^{++}, and has been implicated in cellular necrosis after ischemia. Glutamate levels are increased by ischemia. Experimental blockage of the NMDA receptors during ischemia has resulted in increased hippocampal neuronal survival.

I. After ischemia, blood vessels may become obstructed by large stiff PMNs that adhere to the endothelial cells. Adhesion is mediated by ICAM1 and 2 surface markers on endothelial cells and interleukins on white blood cells. Expression of endothelial cell adhesion molecules is increased by TNF, IFN, and IL-1. The serum levels of these cytokines are increased with ischemia. They enter the circulation 30 minutes after occlusion and reach peak levels in 12 hours. There is increased binding of laminin and fibronectin by PMNs after stroke. New ischemia therapies may be directed toward blocking these factors.

XX. VASCULAR DISEASES

A. Atherosclerosis

1. Plaques consist of eccentric fibrofatty deposits and intimal thickening. The plaques are most common at the ICA origin and the distal basilar artery. They form most likely as a reaction to injury. A subtle intimal injury causes platelet aggregation and endothelial injury increases the permeability to lipoproteins.

2. Macrophages and smooth muscle cells proliferate, accumulate fatty esters, and form lipid-filled foam cells that die and form cholesterol deposits. Initially, the **fatty streak** develops and then a fibrotic cap forms over it. Underlying inflammatory changes ensue with neovascularity and this is followed by hemorrhage, rupture, and ulceration forming a nidus for thrombi and emboli.

3. In evaluating with Doppler ultrasonography, convention is that flow toward the probe is red, away is blue, and nonlaminar flow distal to the stenosis is mixed color. There is normally flow reversal in the distal carotid bulb.

4. Ultrasonography tends to overestimate stenosis and may have difficulty differentiating high-grade stenosis from occlusion.

5. Angiography assesses the degree of stenosis and evaluates for tandem lesions in the carotid siphon and intracranially and for associated vascular lesions such as aneurysms. It helps to determine whether the collateral circulation is adequate to determine whether a shunt will be needed during surgery. Only 20% of the population have a complete circle of Willis. If both the ACA and ACOM fill or the PCA fills, usually a shunt is not needed. Two percent of patients have tandem lesions such as distal stenoses, most frequently in the carotid siphon, but also in the M1 segment of the MCA. These lesions may require angioplasty (**Fig. 194**).

6. There may be atherosclerosis in the aortic arch, proximal subclavian artery, brachiocephalic artery, or vertebral artery.

7. The NASCET study determined that **surgery is beneficial if there are symptomatic lesions with 70 to 99% stenosis**. The percent stenosis is determined by measuring the distal normal ICA diameter and the stenotic diameter: (Distal − stenotic/distal) × 100.

B. Transient ischemic attack (TIA)—the sudden onset of a focal neurologic deficit caused by a vascular lesion lasting < 24 hours. It is usually caused by a platelet-fibrin embolus from an ulcerative atherosclerotic plaque.

C. Reversible ischemic neurologic deficit (RIND) —lasts 24 hours to 1 week.

D. Cerebrovascular accident (CVA) or stroke

1. CVA—the sudden onset of neurologic deficit caused by hemorrhage or ischemia from thrombus, emboli, or hemodynamic alterations.

2. Most strokes are caused by atherosclerosis.

3. Most emboli are either from mural thrombi or valve vegetations. The most common distribution is **MCA** (75%), followed by PCA, and rarely ACA (0.6%).

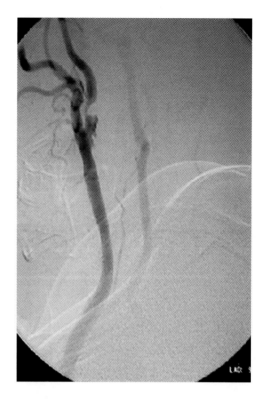

Figure 194   Carotid artery stenosis. Angiogram demonstrates proximal ICA plaque.

4. Death in these patients is most frequently caused by myocardial infarction because of the systemic nature of vascular disease.

5. Angiography after stroke may demonstrate the cause of the stroke. Findings of an infarct are hyperemia or vascular blush in the penumbra from venous luxury perfusion and AV shunting with early draining veins.

6. CT findings (**Fig. 195**)

   (a) Hyperacute phase (< 12 hours)—normal CT (50%), hyperdense MCA with luminal clot (25 to 50%), and obscured lentiform nuclei.

   (b) Acute phase (12 to 24 hours)—decreased density of the basal ganglia and decreased gray/white differentiation at the insula (insular ribbon sign) and cortex.

   (c) 1 to 3 days—mass effect, wedge-shaped low density of the gray and white matter, and possibly hemorrhage.

   (d) 4 to 7 days—gyral enhancement and edema.

   (e) 1 to 8 weeks—enhancement, decreased mass effect, and calcification in children.

   (f) Months—calcifications and encephalomalacia.

7. MRI findings

   (a) Immediate—absence of flow void and intravascular enhancement.

(b) Hyperacute (<12 hours)—hypointense on T1-weighted and hyperintense on T2-weighted MRI.

(c) Acute (12 to 24 hours)—hyperintense on T2-weighted MRI, enhancing meninges adjacent to the stroke, and mass effect.

(d) 1 to 3 days—parenchymal enhancement and hemorrhage.

(e) 4 to 7 days—hemorrhage (25%), increased enhancement, and decreased mass effect.

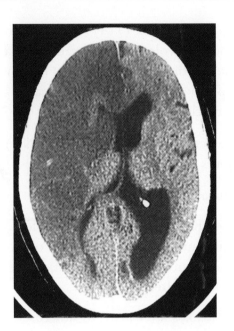

Figure 195   Stroke. Noninfused CT demonstrates right ICA hemispheric hypodensity.

8. Stroke pathology

(a) After 1 hour—axonal changes.

(b) 12 to 24 hours—neuronal necrosis, eosinophilic neurons, neuronal pyknosis.

(c) 24 hours—well-circumscribed necrosis in an arterial territory.

(d) 1 to 2 days—PMNs accumulate.

(e) 2 to 5 days—BBB breakdown, edema, and axon retraction balls at the edge.

(f) 5 to 7 days—gitter cells (lipid-laden macrophages) and neovascularization.

(g) 10 to 20 days—astrocytosis around infarct, rim of gemistocytes.

(h) >3 months—cystic space with fibrillary astrocytes. A 1-cm stroke takes 3 months to become cystic. A stroke tends to preserve the outermost cortical layers unlike a contusion that usually extends to the pia and affects the crests of the gyri.

E. **Pseudolaminar cortical necrosis**—caused by generalized hypoxia, not focal. The middle cortical layers are affected (layers 3, 5, and 6) and there is frequent gyriform hemorrhage.

F. Hemorrhagic stroke—10% of ischemic strokes hemorrhage as a result of reperfusion into areas of brain with damaged blood vessels. Hemorrhage is more common with **emboli** than thrombi. It usually occurs 24 to 48 hours after a stroke. The incidence is higher in large strokes (25%). There is an increased risk of hemorrhage if a hypodensity is detected within 4 hours of a stroke.

G. Lacunar stroke—<1.5 cm, occurs in the basal ganglia, thalamus and white matter, and accounts for 20% of strokes. They are usually caused by hypertension and less commonly by atherosclerosis and thromboemboli. The small arteries are affected by **lipohyalinosis**. The CT is usually negative early on, although the lesion is hypointense on T1-weighted MRI.

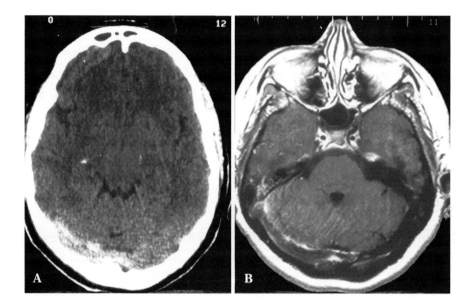

Figure 196 Venous sinus thrombosis. Noninfused CT (A) and T1-weighted MRI (B) demonstrate a thrombosed right transverse sinus.

H. Venous stroke

1. It is more often hemorrhagic and more frequently involves the **white matter** instead of the gray (unlike an arterial stroke). It is frequently secondary to a dural sinus thrombosis.

2. The risk is increased with **dehydration**, **pregnancy**, **infection**, oral contraceptive pills (OCPs), surgery, **hypercoagulable state** (factor V Leiden, protein C and S, and antithrombin III deficiencies), tumor, trauma, drugs, paroxysmal nocturnal hemoglobinuria, lupus anticoagulant, Behçet's syndrome, and inflammatory bowel disease. No cause is identified in 25% of cases.

3. The most frequent sinuses involved in descending order are **superior sagittal sinus**, transverse sinus, sigmoid sinus, and cavernous sinus. Internal cerebrovenous occlusion is rare and causes bilateral deep gray and diencephalic ischemia.

4. Angiogram demonstrates parasagittal collateral venous channels surrounding an empty channel.

5. The CT is hyperdense and may demonstrate an **empty-delta sign** caused by a clot in the transverse sinus (the dural veins become engorged and enhance while the inside of the sinus does not enhance) (**Fig. 196**).

6. **MRV** and/or angiography is the best test for diagnosis.

7. Mortality is 20 to 30%.

I. Pediatric/young adult stroke

1. Accounts for 3% of strokes and is usually caused by congenital heart disease with an embolism. It may also be caused by dissection, infection (syphilis), drugs, OCPs with migraine, coagulation disorder (protein C and S, antithrombin III, or factor 5 Leiden deficiency), Fabry's disease, homocysteinuria, FMD, Marfan's syndrome, collagen vascular disease, ulcerative colitis/Crohn's disease, moyamoya disease, NF1, TS, vasculitis, radiation, and tumors.

2. There is congenital vascular stenosis associated with NF1 and TS.

3. The risk with OCPs is higher if the age is > 35 years or there is tobacco use, hypertension, or migraines. The OCPs also increase the risk of heart disease and SAH. Pregnancy is associated with hemorrhagic stroke secondary to eclampsia, HELLP syndrome, and venous thrombosis.

J. Stroke syndromes

1. Multi-infarct dementia (MID)—distinguish from vasculitis, intravascular lymphoma, hypertensive encephalopathy, and emboli.

2. Locked-in syndrome—the only voluntary motor function preserved is vertical eye movement (in the classic form). It is caused by a large ventral pontine stroke from an occluded basilar artery branch.

3. Weber's syndrome—from a lesion in the midbrain caused by vascular occlusion, tumor, or aneurysm. Findings are oculomotor palsy with crossed hemiplegia. It involves CN III and the corticospinal tract.

4. Benedikt's syndrome—from a lesion in the tegmentum of the midbrain caused by ischemia, hemorrhage, TB, or tumor. Findings are oculomotor palsy with contralateral hemiplegia and cerebellar ataxia and tremor. It involves CN III, the red nucleus, corticospinal tract, and brachium conjunctivum.

5. Millard-Gubler syndrome—form a lesion in the pons. Findings are facial and abducens palsies with contralateral hemiplegia. It is caused by ischemia or tumor and involves CNs VI, VII, and the corticospinal tract.

6. **Wallenberg's syndrome** (lateral medullary syndrome)—from a lesion in the lateral tegmentum of the medulla. Findings are ipsilateral CN V, IX (decreased gag and taste), X (dysphagia and hoarseness), and XI palsies, Horner's syndrome, cerebellar ataxia, hiccups, nystagmus, and contralateral loss of pain and temperature sense. It is caused by vertebral artery (more common) or PICA occlusion usually by thrombosis of the artery secondary to an atherosclerotic plaque but occasionally caused by embolism or dissection. It involves the spinal nucleus and tract of CNS V, CNs IX, X, and XI; lateral spinothalamic tract; descending sympathetic fibers; and the inferior peduncle (spinocerebellar and olivocerebellar tracts) (**Fig. 197**).

7. Medial medullary syndrome—from a lesion in the medial medulla. Findings are ipsilateral tongue paralysis, and contralateral paralysis of upper and lower extremities (spares face) and decreased body touch and proprioception. It is caused by vertebral artery or branch of lower basilar occlusion. It involves **CN XII**, **pyramidal tract**, and **medial lemniscus**.

8. Subclavian steal—**proximal** subclavian artery stenosis (proximal to the origin of the vertebral artery) with reversal of flow in the vertebral artery to the upper limb. There is a noticeable pulse difference between the two upper limbs (**Fig. 198**).

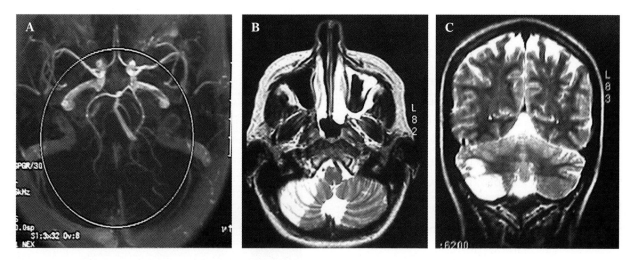

Figure 197   Stroke. MRA (A) demonstrating absence of right vertebral artery flow and axial (B) and coronal (C) T2-weighted MRIs demonstrating right PICA distribution CVA (from vertebral artery occlusion).

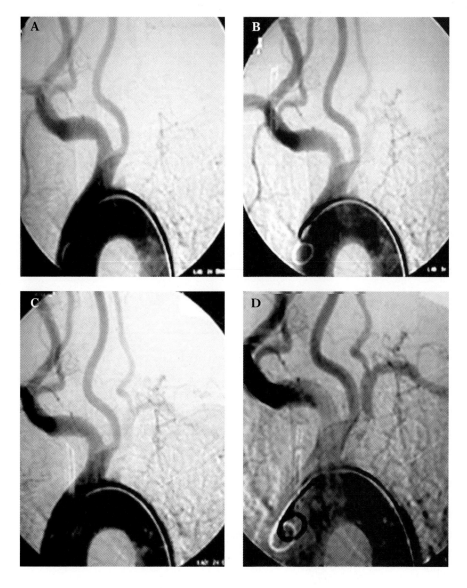

Figure 198   Subclavian steal. Serial angiograms (A to D) demonstrate proximal left subclavian artery stenosis with retrograde filling from the left vertebral artery. A bovine variant with the left ICA originating from the brachiocephalic trunk is also demonstrated.

K. Stroke-related diseases

    1. Moyamoya disease

       (a) Idiopathic progressive arteriopathy of childhood, with unknown cause. It is more frequent in Japan. It causes progressive stenosis or occlusion of the **distal ICA** and proximal ACA and MCA.

       (b) Multiple parenchymal, leptomeningeal, and transdural collaterals develop.

       (c) Angiogram demonstrates enlarged lenticulostriate, thalamoperforate, and collateral vessels forming a **"puff of smoke."** Eighty percent of patients develop stroke and 50% have atrophy, especially in the anterior circulation (**Fig. 199**). A similar vascular pattern may be seen with any progressive occlusive vascular disease (radiation, atherosclerosis, and sickle cell disease).

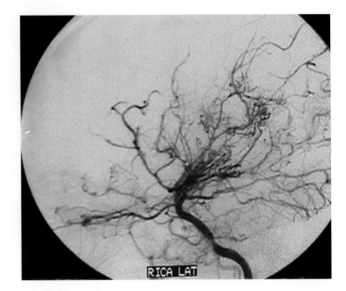

Figure 199   Moyamoya disease. Angiogram demonstrates distal ICA occlusion with prominent leptomenigeal collaterals "puff of smoke."

       (d) In children it presents with **transient weakness** and in adults with SAH.

       (e) Pathologic examination demonstrates intimal thickening and fibrotic changes. Moyamoya disease is associated with Down syndrome.

    2. Sickle cell anemia—6 to 9% of patients have strokes that are usually ischemic. There are occlusions of small and large vessels and multiple aneurysms in unusual locations. There is endothelial injury caused by adhesions of sickle cells followed by vascular degeneration and sometimes aneurysm formation.

    3. Marfan's syndrome and homocysteinuria—cause large vessel vasculopathy, coagulopathy, and subluxation of lenses.

    4. Ehlers-Danlos syndrome—vascular fragility associated with carotid-cavernous fistulas and arterial narrowing.

    5. NFI—associated with aortic, celiac, mesenteric, and renal vascular stenosis, and cerebrovascular stenosis, aneurysms, AVMs, and moyamoya disease. There are no vascular abnormalities associated with NF2.

    6. Tuberous sclerosis—associated with stenoses and aneurysms (especially the thoracic abdominal aorta).

    7. Klippel-Trénaunay-Weber syndrome—associated with aneurysms and carotid aplasia.

    8. Menke's kinky hair disease—associated with tortuous abdominal, visceral, and intracranial arteries.

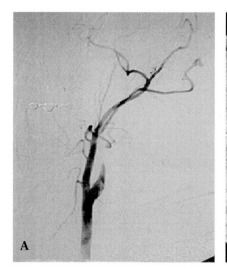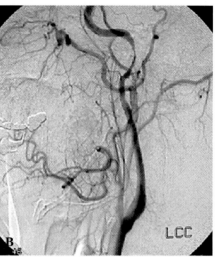

Figure 200   Carotid artery dissection. Angiograms demonstrate (A) cervical ICA and (B) petrous ICA tapered narrowings.

9. Fibromuscolar disease (FMD)—a segmental noninflammatory narrowing of blood vessels by intimal or medial proliferation. It most commonly affects the **cervical ICA** (75%), vertebral artery (25%), and renal arteries. 75% are bilateral. There is a female predominance and it develops before 50 years. Angiogram has a **"string of beads"** appearance. 20% are associated with an intracranial aneurysm and they are also associated with dissections, AVMs and emboli. It is believed to be caused by degeneration of elastic tissue with loss of muscle and accumulation of fibrous tissue. The segmental dilations are caused by atrophy of the vessel wall. Treatment if there is a stroke may be with endovascular dilation or excision of an affected segment with reconstruction (see Fig. 211).

10. Radiation vasculopathy—causes gradual narrowing and occlusion that occurs usually after 18 months.

11. Dissection of the ICA

    (a) It may cause a sudden onset of nonthrobbing ipsilateral head and neck pain, Horner's syndrome, peripheral neuropathy of CNs X, XI, or XII (by occlusion of arterial feeders), and focal ischemic symptoms.

    (b) Risk is increased with trauma, FMD, cystic medial necrosis, hypertension, migraine, drugs, OCPs, pharyngeal infections, vasculopathy, Marfan's syndrome, and homocysteinuria.

    (c) Evaluation is with MRI/MRA and angiogram that demonstrates a **string sign** or occlusion (**Fig. 200**).

    (d) The dissection spares the carotid bulb and usually starts **2 cm above the carotid bifurcation**. It less frequently involves the supraclinoid ICA and the proximal ACA or MCA.

    (e) Treatment is with anticoagulation. Without stroke, 85% do well. With stroke, 25% mortality is present and 50% are permanently impaired.

12. Dissection of the vertebral artery—usually occurs at the segment **between C2 and the occiput**. See Chapter 5 for more detail on dissections (**Fig. 201**).

13. Extrinsic compressive lesions—tumor, osteophytes, fibrous bands, and infection.

14. Raeder's syndrome—causes unilateral headache and face pain of the V1 and 2 distributions and Horner's syndrome. The ICA may be narrowed by sinusitis, arteritis, or dissection.

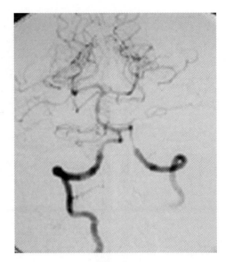

Figure 201   Vertebral artery dissection. Angiogram demonstrates left distal vertebral artery narrowing.

L. Vasculitis

1. Infectious vasculitis—caused by *H. influenza* (common cause of stroke in children), TB, *Actinomyces* (directly invades vessel wall), herpes encephalitis, and syphilis (MCA distribution gummas and diffuse involvement of cortical arteries and veins). There is inflammation in the vessel wall with necrosis, occlusion, stroke, or hemorrhage. Endocarditis has a 5 to 10% risk of SAH as a result of mycotic aneurysms, stroke, or focal vasculitis. Encephalitis is rarely hemorrhagic, except with HSV2.

2. Immune complex vasculitis

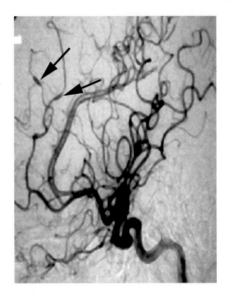

Figure 202   Lupus vasculitis. Angiogram demonstrates multiple distal ACA fusiform dilations (arrows) and narrowings.

(a) Polyarteritis nodosa—the most common necrotic vasculitis with CNS lesions. It affects small and medium-sized arteries throughout the body. It causes polyneuropathy that may be symmetric or asymmetric (**mononeuropathy multiplex**) by obliteration of the vaso nervorum, and is associated with microaneurysms (70%), stenosis, and thrombosis. It also causes skin purpura and renal dysfunction.

(b) Systemic lupus erythematosus (SLE)—an autoimmune disease caused by **antinuclear antibodies**. 75% of cases involve the CNS. 50% of cases develop stroke mainly caused by antiphospholipid antibodies, coagulopathy (with hemorrhage), and cardiac valve disease (Libman-Sacks endocarditis). Vasculitis is rare. It may also cause myelopathy or peripheral neuropathy. There is frequently a malar butterfly rash. Treatment is with steroids (**Fig. 202**).

(c) Others—allergic angiitis, serum sickness, and other collagen vascular diseases.

3. Cell-mediated vasculitis

   (a) Temporal arteritis

   (i)   A subacute granulomatous inflammation with **giant cells**. Peak age is 70 years. It affects **extracranial vessels** (especially the temporal branches of the ECA).

   (ii) It is an autoimmune disease with mononuclear cell inflammation of all three layers with multinucleated giant cells and resorption of the internal elastic lamina. There may be antibodies to the external elastic lamina.

   (iii) Skip lesions are common so that segments of abnormal artery are interspersed with unaffected segments.

   (iv) Symptoms include low-grade fever, weight loss, headache, local tenderness, **elevated ESR**, and occasionally polymyalgia rheumatica with proximal muscle pain. The **ophthalmic artery** may be involved, but never intracranial vessels.

   (v)   Treatment is with low-dose **steroids** to decrease the risk of blindness.

   (b) Takayasu arteritis—occlusive thromboaortopathy with giant cell arteritis affecting the aorta and its branches and the pulmonary arteries causing stenosis and aneurysms. It most commonly occurs in young Oriental females. Symptoms include fever, weight loss, elevated ESR, and decreased peripheral pulses (**pulseless disease**). There may be visual loss. Treatment is with steroids and revascularization.

   (c) Wegener's granulomatosis—occurs in adults with male predominance. It involves respiratory, renal, and CNS vessels and causes peripheral and cranial neuropathies. It is due to **antineutrophil antibodies** and is treated with cyclophosphamide.

4. Chemical vasculitis—caused by ergots, pseudoephedrine, amphetamine, and OCPs (especially with tobacco use).

5. Other causes of vasculitis

   (a) Sarcoid

   (b) Kawasaki's disease (mucocutaneous lymph node syndrome)—fusiform ectasia and aneurysms.

   (c) Buerger's disease (thromboangiitis obliterans)—affects small and medium-sized arteries and veins and is associated with tobacco use.

   (d) Behçet disease—a recurrent inflammatory disease with male predominance that affects arteries and veins. It is most common in Japan and the Mediteranean. It is associated with oral and genital ulcers, uveitis, ulcerative colitis, erythema nodosum, polyarthritis, arterial occlusions, aneuryms, and thrombophlebitis. There may be brain stem, meningoencephalitic or organic confusional syndromes. The CNS is involved in 10 to 45% of patients. Treatment is with steroids.

   (e) Thrombotic thrombocytopenic purpura (TTP) affects young adults and involves small vessels. It causes fever, thrombocytopenia, anemia, and renal and hepatic dysfunction, and leads to hemorrhages in the body and stroke in the brain.

M. Hypertension

1. Acute hypertension—causes increased pinocytosis in the cerebral capillaries and arterioles with BBB breakdown, fibrin deposition around blood vessels, brain swelling and edema, and increased ICP.

2. Chronic hypertension

   (a) It causes serum proteins to accumulate in the basement membrane and causes collagen deposition, medial hyalination, loss of muscularis layer, vessel dilation or stenosis, and occasionally fatty macrophage accumulation (lipohyalinosis) in small muscular arteries.

   (b) It most commonly affects the basal ganglia, pons, centrum semiovale, and cerebellum.

   (c) Charcot-Bouchard aneurysms form on the lenticulostriate arteries. There are dilated perivascular spaces, état lacunaire (in the centrum semiovale) and état criblé (in the basal ganglia), which form lacunae with gliosis but no symptoms.

   (d) Hemorrhage may be caused by rupture of Charcot-Bouchard aneurysms or by occlusion and secondary rupture of small penetrating arteries.

3. Hypertensive encephalopathy

   (a) Extreme hypertension causes **loss of autoregulation** with vasospasm, dilation, BBB breakdown, and edema.

   (b) Lesions form in the external capsule, basal ganglia, gray-white junction, and occipital lobe (more in the posterior circulation because there is less sympathetic input).

   (c) Symptoms include headaches, seizures, obtundation, and focal deficits, as well as manifestations of other end organ damage such as renal and cardiac disease.

   (d) Hypertensive encephalopathy usually occurs with toxemia, pre-eclampsia/eclampsia, chronic renal failure, TTP, hemolytic uremic syndrome, SLE, and renovascular hypertension.

4. **Binswanger's disease**—causes hypertension and dementia with lacunae or demyelination in the centrum semiovale with arteriolar sclerosis.

5. Pre-eclampsia—hypertension and proteinuria that develops after 24 weeks of pregnancy. It occurs in 5 to 10% of pregnancies. Eclampsia is present when seizures or coma develop. It occurs in 0.1% of pregnancies, is fatal in 13%, and is associated with deep hemorrhages and white matter changes on MRI.

N. Intraparenchymal hemorrhage (IPH)

1. Etiologies—hypertension, amyloid angiopathy, tumor, AVMs, vasculitis, and coagulopathy.

2. CT appearance

   (a) Acute—the clot is hyperdense because of increased hemoglobin (Hb) and proteins. It may be hypodense if there is unretracted liquid clot, active bleeding, a coagulation disorder, or a hematocrit < 30.

   (b) Subacute (1 to 6 weeks)—isodense.

      (c) Chronic—hypodense.

      (d) Residua—hypodense (37%), slit lesion (25%), calcification (10%), or no abnormality (27%).

3. MRI appearance

      (a) **Hyperacute** (few hours)—contains oxyHb, isointense T1 and hyperintense T2.

      (b) **Acute**—contains deoxyHb, hypo or iso T1 and hypoT2.

      (c) **Subacute** (days to months)—contains metHb, intracellular (3 to 14 days) hyperT1 and hypoT2, and extracellular (>2 weeks) hyperT1 and T2.

      (d) **Chronic**—contains ferritin and hemosiderin, isoT1 and hypo T2.

      (e) Nonparamagnetic heme—hypoT1 and hyperT2.

      (f) **Rim of hemosiderin**—hypoT1 and 2.

      (g) The clot interior is hypoxic and this may delay the Hb denaturation.

4. Hypertensive intra–parenohymal hemorrage (IPH)

      (a) The most common cause of nontraumatic intracranial hemorrhage. Avarage age is younger than the thrombotic stroke group. There is no sex predominance, and in the United States, African-Americans are affected more than Caucasians.

      (b) It is due to **Charcot-Bouchard aneurysms** or lipohyalinosis of the penetrating arterioles of the brain. Locations are **putamen** (60%), thalamus (20%), pons (10%), cerebellum (near the dentate, 5%), and subcortical white matter (2%). The clot extends to the ventricle in 50% of cases and this carries a worse prognosis (**Fig. 203**).

      (c) Overall mortality is 25% and is related mainly to the size of the hemorrhage.

      (d) Lobar hemorrhages are more likely due to **amyloid angiopathy** in the elderly. Putamenal hemorrhages cause weakness by compression of the IC and eye deviation toward the lesion. Thalamic hemorrhages cause weakness, sensory loss, and ocular dysfunction (**persistent down-gaze**). Cerebellar hemorrhages cause eye deviation away from the lesion and ocular bobbing. Pontine lesions cause fixed pinpoint pupils.

      (e) Surgery may be beneficial for lesions >3 cm in the cerebellum, but has not proven helpful for puntamen or thalamus hemorrhages.

5. Amyloid angiopathy (congophilic)

      (a) It usually occurs after 70 years of age and is the most common cause of intracranial hemorrhage in the normotensive elderly. It occasionally occurs in younger patients if of the familial variety (in the Netherlands and Iceland).

      (b) The contractile elements in the media of the arteries and arterioles of the leptomeningeal and superficial cortical vessels are replaced by noncontractile amyloid b-protein with a β-pleated sheet configuration. Blood vessels become dilated with thick walls containing pink amorphous material. They may form aneurysms.

      (c) The amyloid is yellow-green with dichromism/**birefringence when stained with Congo red dye and viewed under polarized light (Fig. 204).**

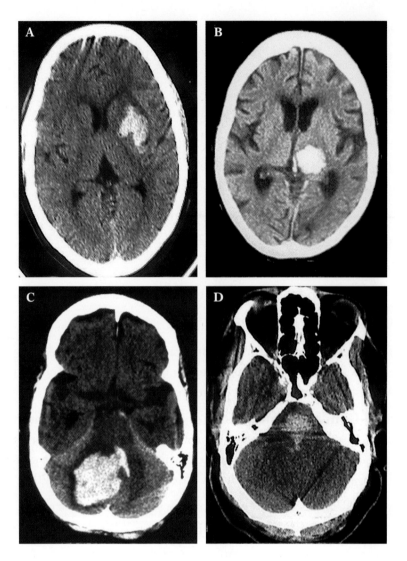

Figure 203   Hypertensive intraparenchymal hemorrhage. Noninfused CTs demonstrate (A) putamen, (B) thalamus, (C) cerebellum, and (D) pons hemorrhages.

(d) The major protein is amyloid β peptide (although it is the cystatin C variant in the hereditary type).

(e) Amyloid angiopathy causes multiple lobar hemorrhages in the centrum semiovale that often extend to the subarachnoid space. These vessel changes also are seen with Down syndrome, Alzheimer's disease, spongiform encephalitis, radiation necrosis, and vasculitis.

6. Drugs—50% of drug-related hemorrhages are spontaneous and 50% are associated with an AVM or aneurysm. Manifestations may include stroke, venous occlusion, abscess, vasculitis, and mycotic aneurysms. Cocaine enhances platelet aggregation and spasm and may cause ischemic strokes. Amphetamines directly irritate the vessel wall and cause vasculitis.

7. Blood dyscrasias—15% of nontraumatic nonaneurysmal intracranial hemorrhages (ICHs) are caused by anticoagulant therapy. One percent of patients with MI treated with thrombolytics have ICH develop. This complication carries a 60% mortality.

8. Germinal matrix hemorrhages

   (a) They occur in **premature infants**.

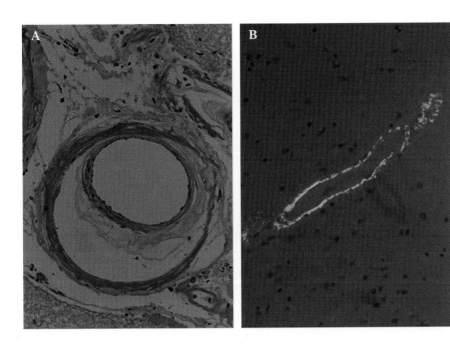

Figure 204   Amyloid angiopathy. (A) H and E stain demonstrating amyloid deposition within the vessel wall; (B) Congo red stain demonstrating negative birefringence in polarized light.

(b) The germinal matrix consists of thin-walled vessels and proliferating cells in the subependymal zone and it normally involutes at 36 weeks' gestational age.

(c) The blood supply is from the lenticulostriate arteries, choroidal arteries, and the artery of Heubner. It typically hemorrhages **a few days after a premature birth** because of hypoxia/ischemia in the deep **watershed zone** that supplies the germinal matrix.

(d) In full-term births, the most common location of intracranial hemorrhage is intraventricular hemorrhage from the choroid plexus.

(e) Germinal matrix hemorrhage grades

    (i)   Grade 1—limited to the germinal matrix.

    (ii)   Grade 2—blood in the ventricle, but no increase in ventricular size.

    (iii) Grade 3—blood in the ventricle with hydrocephalus.

    (iv) Grade 4—intraparenchymal extension of the hemorrhage.

9.   Hemorrhage with malignancies

(a) There is increased incidence with coagulopathy and chemotherapy.

(b) The cause may be neovascularization, necrosis, plasminogen activators, or direct vessel invasion. It occurs in 1 to 15% of tumors.

(c) The most commonly hemorrhagic primary tumors are high-grade astrocytoma, oligodendroglioma, pituitary adenoma, hemangioblastoma, lymphoma, sarcoma, ependymoma, schwannoma, epidermoid, PNET, choroid plexus papilloma, and teratoma.

(d) The most commonly hemorrhagic metastatic tumors are **choriocarcinoma**, melanoma, and renal cell carcinoma. Hemorrhage is detected in 15% of metastatic brain tumors.

(e) Arachnoid cysts may hemorrhage and are associated with SDH.

O. Aneurysms

    1. The rupture of cerebral aneurysms accounts for 85% of nontraumatic SAH (15% AVM and 5% arterial dissection). Ninety percent of the blood is cleared from the CSF in 1 week. The MRI is better than CT for detecting subacute and chronic SAH. Repeated SAH or IVH may cause hemosiderin and ferritin to deposit over the leptomeninges and brain (superficial siderosis) and manifest with cerebellar dysfunction, long tract signs, and impaired hearing.

    2. Saccular aneurysms

        (a) The most common type of aneurysm. Peak age at rupture is 40 to 60 years with a female predominance.

        (b) They usually occur at the arterial bifurcations at the base of the brain. Ninety percent are in the anterior circulation (PCOM 30%, ACOM 30%, MCA 20%, and ICA) and 10% are in the posterior circulation (basilar apex 5%, SCA, VBJ, PICA, and rarely AICA) (**Figs. 205 through 222**).

        (c) The risk of rupture is probably related to size and location. In multiple aneurysm cases the site of the ruptured aneurysm can be predicted by aneurysm location, irregular shape, daughter loculus, surrounding clot, more proximal location, and focal spasm. Aneurysms are multiple in 20% of cases.

        (d) Risk factors include female sex, age, hypertension, atherosclerosis, FMD (20 to 50% have aneurysms), Marfan's syndrome, Ehler-Danlos syndrome, polycystic kidney disease, coarctation of the aorta, high flow state (AVM), and familial history.

        (e) They were originally thought to be congenital and caused by medial defects of the elastic lamina at the vessel bifurcations, but now are thought to be acquired from hemodynamically induced vascular injury because they rarely are seen before 20 years.

        (f) Pathologic examination reveals deterioration of the internal elastic lamina and muscularis at the junction of the vessel and the aneurysm.

        (g) In children, they are rare, more common in males, larger, in unusual locations, and frequently associated with trauma and infection.

        (h) Rehemorrhage rate is highest in the first 24 hours, 20% in 2 weeks, 50% in 6 months, and 3% per year after that. The hemorrhage risk is 1 to 2% per year if unruptured (although if it is <10 mm, the rate is 0.05% per year).

        (i) The long-term outcome after hemorrhage in patients who survive to reach the hospital is death (25%), impairment (15%), and normal (60%).

        (j) Angiography—used to assess spasm, collateral supply, filling vessels, and the relationship of the aneurysm to the parent vessel and perforators.

        (k) Giant aneurysms (>2.5 cm)—may or may not have a lower hemorrhage rate. They bleed into themselves from the wall, contain multilayered clots, and have a thick fibrous wall. They more frequently cause symptoms by mass effect.

        (l) Classical SAH locations—frontal horn (anterior choroidal), interhemispheric fissure (ACOM), sylvian fissure (MCA), and fourth ventricle (posterior circulation) (**Fig. 223**).

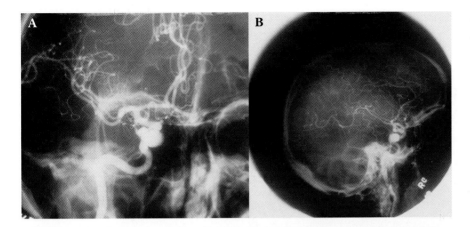

Figure 205   Cavernous ICA aneurysm. AP (A) and lateral (B) angiograms.

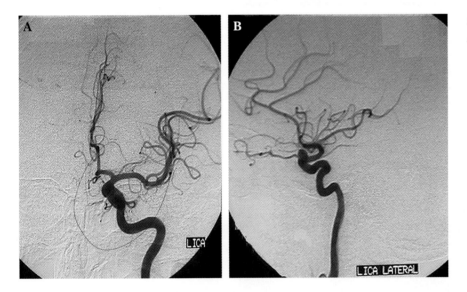

Figure 206   Ophthalmic ICA aneurysm. AP (A) and lateral (B) angiograms.

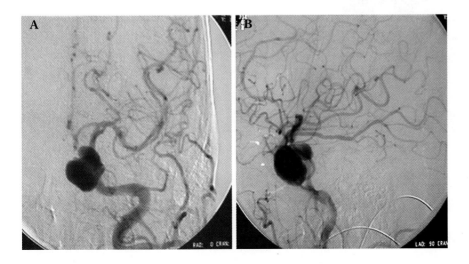

Figure 207   Giant ophthalmic ICA aneurysm. AP (A) and lateral (B) angiograms.

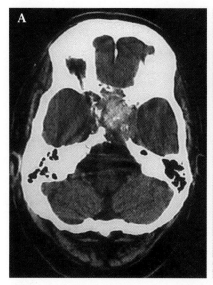
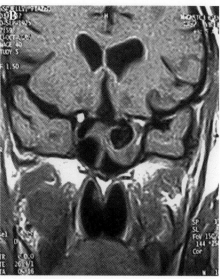

Figure 208   Giant ophthalmic ICA aneurysm. Axial CT (A) and coronal T1-weighted MRI (B) demonstrate erosive mass with partial thrombus and flow void.

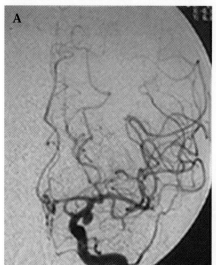
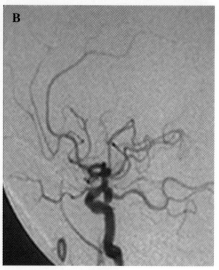

Figure 209   PCOM artery aneurysm. AP (A) and lateral (B) angiograms.

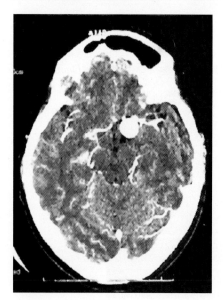

Figure 210   PCOM artery aneurysm. Infused axial CT demonstrates left-sided mass.

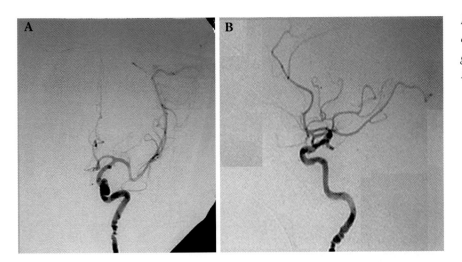

Figure 211   Anterior choroidal artery aneurysm. AP (A) and lateral (B) angiograms. There is also FMD in the cervical ICA.

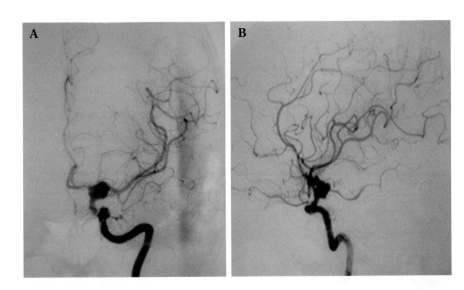

Figure 212   ICA bifurcation aneurysm. AP (A) and lateral (B) angiograms.

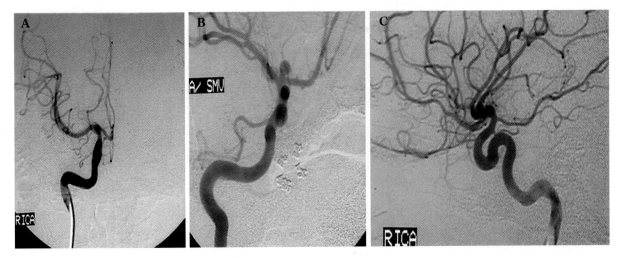

Figure 213   ICA bifurcation aneurysm. AP (A), oblique (B), and lateral (C) angiograms. Note the double density at the bifurcation on the AP view.

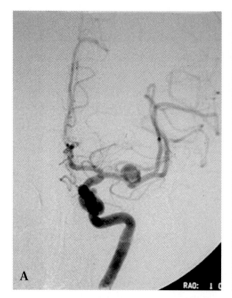
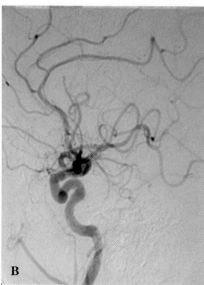

Figure 214   MCA aneurysm. AP (A) and lateral (B) angiograms.

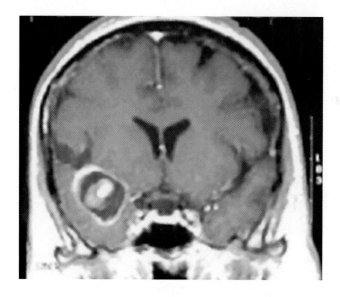

Figure 215   Giant MCA aneurysm. Coronal T1-weighted MRI with gadolinium infusion demonstrating right-sided lesion partially filled with thrombus.

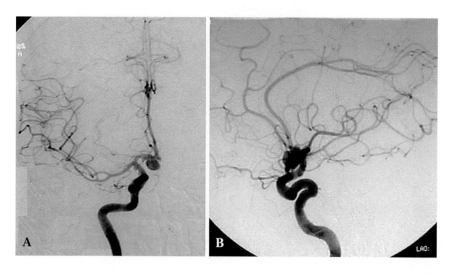

Figure 216   ACOM artery aneurysm. AP (A) and lateral (B) angiograms.

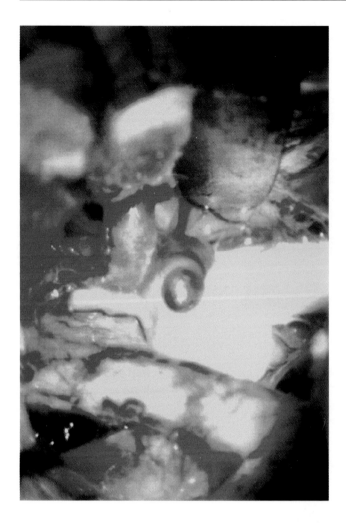

Figure 217   ACOM aneurysm. Aneurysm pointing anteriorly.

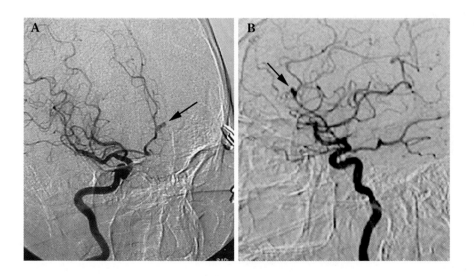

Figure 218   Distal ACA aneurysm. AP (A) and lateral (B) angiograms.

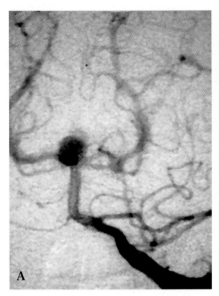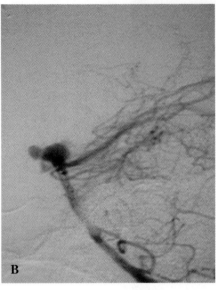

Figure 219   Basilar artery apex aneurym. AP (A) and lateral (B) angiograms.

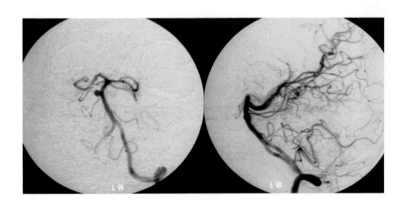

Figure 220   AICA aneurysm. AP (A) and lateral (B) angiograms.

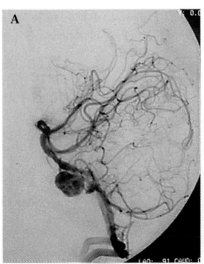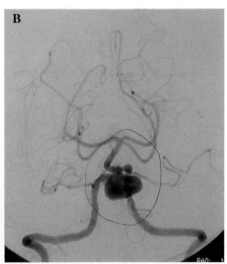

Figure 221   Vertebrobasilar junction aneurysm. Lateral (A) and AP (B) angiograms.

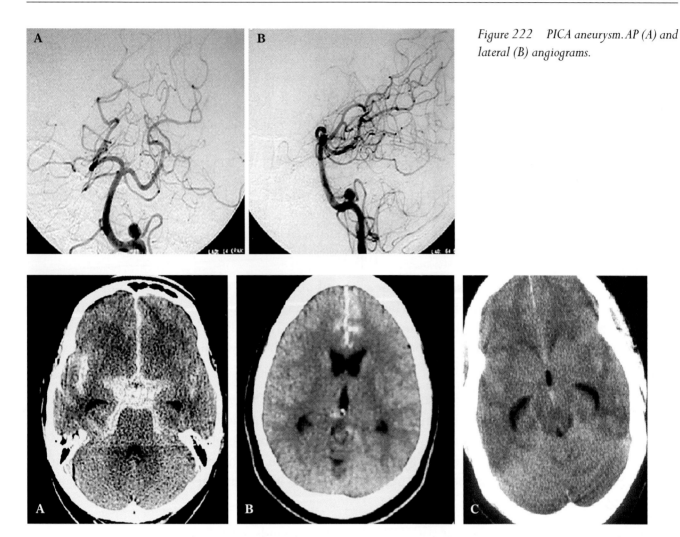

Figure 222   PICA aneurysm. AP (A) and lateral (B) angiograms.

Figure 223   Subarachnoid hemorrhage. Noninfused axial CTs of (A) suprasellar cistern hemorrhage from a ruptured PCOM aneurysm, (B) interhemispheric hemorrhage from a ruptured ACOM aneurysm, and (C) interpeduncular cistern hemorrhage from a ruptured basilar apex aneurysm.

(m) Complications of aneurysmal SAH—**vasospasm** (angiographic in 30 to 70% and symptomatic in 20 to 30%, 50% of these patients die or suffer permanent deficits, peak time is 4 to 14 days), rehemorrhage (20% in 2 weeks if not treated, occurs in 8 to 12% of patients), hydrocephalus, edema, and stroke (**Fig. 224**).

(n) Aneurysmal SAH is associated with fever, ECG changes (possibly by hypothalamic ischemia with sympathetic dysfunction), and preretinal subhyaloid hemorrhages.

(o) In 15% of SAH, no aneurysm is demonstrated. If the angiogram is repeated in 2 weeks, 20% of these reveal an aneurysm.

(p) Treatment options are surgical clipping, wrapping, and trapping and endovascular coiling. Operative mortality is 3%.

(q) If the aneurysm is unruptured and < 10 mm, consider repeat imaging every year. Consider intervention if it enlarges.

(r) **Infundibulum**—a funnel-shaped dilation at the origin of a vessel, is < 3 to 4 mm wide, with a vessel exiting from the apex of the funnel. It probably is caused by incomplete regression of the vessel during fetal development. They are most common at the origin of the PCOM from the ICA but occasionally occur on other arteries.

(s) **Benign perimesencephalic hemorrhage**—located in the interpeduncular and ambient cisterns, seldom rehemorrhages, has a good prognosis, and is postulated to be caused by the rupture of small pontine and perimesencephlic veins (**Fig. 225**).

3. Fusiform aneurysms—caused by atherosclerosis, infection (syphilis), and vasculitis. They form when damage to the media causes the artery to elongate. They are most common in older patients and in the posterior circulation. Symptoms are caused by stroke, thrombus with mass effect, or hemorrhage (**Fig. 226**).

4. Mycotic aneurysms—caused by an infected embolism to the intima or vaso vasorum and account for 2 to 3% of aneurysms. The thoracic aorta is the most frequent site, and the most common intracranial location is the **distal MCA territory**. They are usually multiple and are caused by bacteria or fungi. Ten percent of patients with SBE will develop a mycotic aneurysm (**Fig. 227**).

5. Dissecting aneurysms—more commonly extracranial and tends to spare the CCA and carotid bulb. They usually involve the midcervical and petrous ICA, and in the vertebral artery occur from C2 to the occiput. They are caused by trauma, infection, cystic medial necrosis, and FMD. Blood accumulates in the vessel wall by means of a tear in the intima and internal elastic lamina. Subintimal accumulation may cause occlusion, whereas subadventitial accumulation may cause an aneurysm and hemorrhage.

6. Traumatic aneurysms—occur with 50% of gunshot wounds to the head and are usually pseudoaneurysms. With nonpenetrating trauma they are usually on the distal ACA. Suspicion should be raised if there is abundant SAH in head injury, after penetrating head injury, or with late bleeding after head injury.

7. Oncotic aneurysms—occur with left atrial myxoma and choriocarcinoma.

8. Flow-related aneuryms—occur with AVMs (2.7 to 30%) and are usually located on the proximal or distal feeding vessels. There is no increased hemorrhage risk with proximal arterial feeder aneurysms, although the risk is increased with a nidus aneurysm (10% hemorrhage). They are thin-walled, have arterial pressure, and frequently hemorrhage.

9. True aneurysms—involve all three layers (intima, media, and adventitia). False aneurysms have no media or internal elastic lamina. Pseudoaneurysms are recanalized blood clots and have no wall besides the clot. Cerebral aneurysms are usually false.

P. Vascular malformations

1. They are congenital and arise in the fetus during vessel development. Only AVMs and cavernous malformations have a clinically important hemorrhage risk.

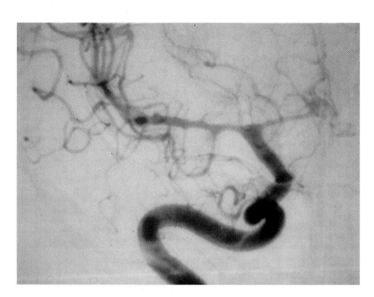

Figure 224   Vasospasm. Right ICA angiogram with narrowing of the proximal ACA and MCA.

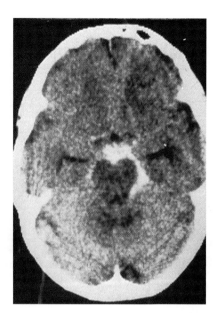

Figure 225   Benign perimesencephalic hemorrhage. CT demonstrates typical SAH extending into the left ambient cistern (angiogram was normal).

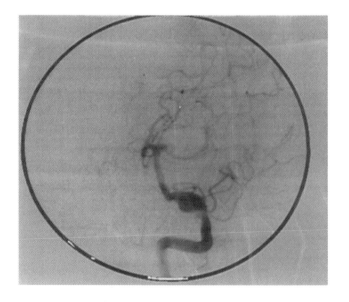

Figure 226   Fusiform aneurysm. Oblique vertebral artery angiogram with left distal vertebral fusiform aneurysm.

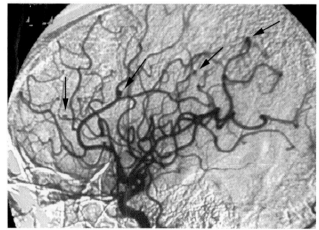

Figure 227   Mycotic (infectious) aneurysms. Angiogram demonstrates multiple distal anterior circulation aneurysms (arrows).

2. Arteriovenous malformations (AVMs)

    (a) Peak age at presentation is 20 to 40 years and there is no gender predilection. Twenty-five percent occur before 15 years and they are 1/10 as common as aneurysms.

    (b) They are composed of thin-walled and thick-walled channels connecting arteries to veins without intervening capillary beds. Ninety percent are hemispheric and 15% are in the posterior fossa. They are frequently cone shaped, extending from the subpial surface with the apex at the ventricle.

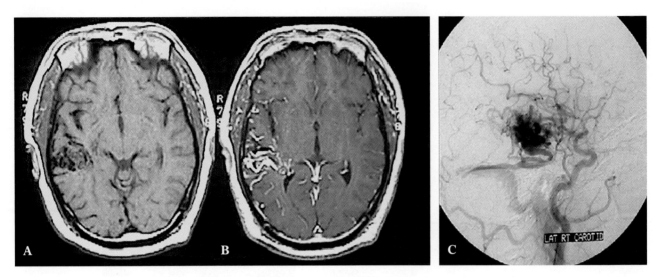

Figure 228   *AVM. Axial T1-weighted MRI noninfused (A) and infused (B) demonstrating serpentine vessels and angiogram (C) demonstrating early draining veins and AVM nidus.*

(c) CT—demonstrates **serpiginous vessels** and calcifications (30%). MRI demonstrates blood in different stages and flow voids.

(d) Angiogram—demonstrates **early draining veins** (also seen with stroke, luxury perfusion, tumors, contusions, postictal, and infection). An aneurysm is found on the feeding vessel or nidus in 8–12% of cases (**Figs. 228 through 230**).

(e) "Cryptic" AVMs—not detected by angiogram, in some cases because the feeding vessels are occluded by thrombus.

(f) Vascular steal causes local ischemia and atrophy. The adjacent brain has ischemic changes, surrounding gliosis, hemosiderin-laden macrophages, and calcifications. **There usually is no intervening normal brain.**

(g) They are developmental but may increase, decrease, or not change in size spontaneously over time.

(h) Symptoms—hemorrhage (50%, mixed SAH and parenchymal), seizures (25%), headaches (20%), and focal symptoms (15%). A bruit may be heard in 25%.

(i) Hemorrhage risk—2 to 4% per year. Rehemorrhage risk is 6% for the first 6 months and then 3% per year. Each hemorrhage carries a 10% mortality and 25% morbidity. There is increased risk of hemorrhage if they are small, have deep drainage, are periventricular, or have an intranidal aneurysm. Ninety-eight percent are solitary, if multiple consider Wyburn-Mason and ROW syndromes.

(j) Surgery. See Section VI—mortality of 1.3% and morbidity of 7.8% but depends highly on case selection.

(k) Radiation—an option if the AVM diameter is < 3 cm (85% 2-year occlusion, but risk of hemorrhage may be increased up to 10.5% in the 2 years until the AVM is obliterated).

(l) Endovascular embolization—helpful surgical adjuvant but is seldom effective by itself in the long term, except for small AVMs that can be completely obliterated by glue embolization.

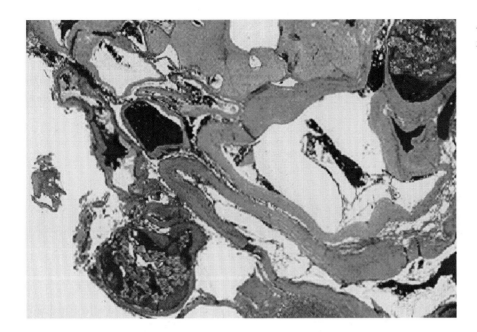

Figure 229   AVM (H and E). Multiple irregular thick and thin-walled vessels.

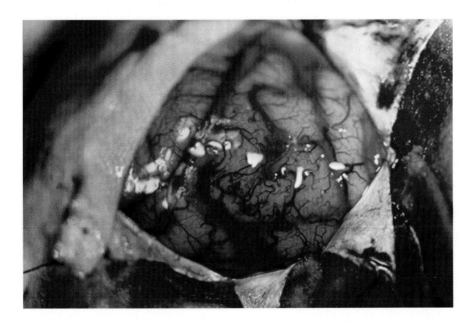

Figure 230   AVM. Arterialized cortical veins.

3. Vein of Galen aneurysm/malformation

    (a) Presentations—in the neonate with **cyanotic heart disease**, in the infant with **hydrocephalus and seizures**, and in children with **SAH**.

    (b) Type 1—the most common, is present at birth, and is associated with high-output heart failure and hydrocephalus. It is an arterio-venous fistula (AVF) of the anterior and posterior choroidal arteries to the median venous sac (embryonal precursor of the vein of Galen).

    (c) Type 2—occurs in older infants, causes developmental delay and ocular symptoms, and is a parenchymal AVM in the thalamus/midbrain with thalamoperforate feeders draining into the vein of Galen. Occasionally, there is thrombosis of the venous sac (**Fig. 231**).

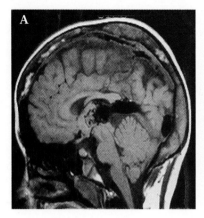
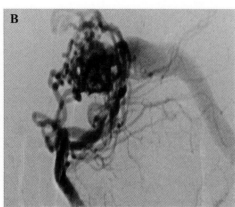

Figure 231   Vein of Galen malformation. Sagittal T1-weighted MRI (A) with diencephalic serpentine vessels and an enlarged vein of Galen, and lateral basilar artery angiogram (B) with early filling of vein of Galen system.

4. Dural AVM's

   (a) There is **no discrete nidus** and the feeding vessels are usually in the wall of a dural venous sinus. They are **acquired** (not congenital) after **dural thrombosis** and recanalization with microfistula formation. The peakage at presentation is 40–60 years.

   (b) The **transverse and sigmoid sinuses** are the most common sites followed by the cavernous sinus and rarely the superior sagittal or straight sinus. Seven percent are multiple. They account for 10 to 15% of AVMs and up to 30% of posterior fossa AVMs.

   (c) Symptoms are bruit and headache (if sigmoid or transverse) and proptosis, chemosis, ophthalmoplegia, and bruit (if cavernous).

   (d) If the dural AVM drains forward into the sinus; it rarely hemorrhages. If there is **reflux flow into the cortical veins**, there is a higher incidence of SAH and IPH. They may also cause venous ischemia and communicating hydrocephalus from venous congestion.

   (e) Feeders usually are from the **ECA circulation** (occipital or meningeal arteries) and occasionally from the tentorial and dural ICA and vertebral artery branches. There is frequent sinus occlusion.

   (f) Traumatic cavernous carotid fistula (**CCF)** usually has one feeder. Spontaneous CCF has multiple feeders and usually occurs in middle-aged females.

   (g) CT demonstrates a dilated superior ophthalmic vein in CCF. MRI demonstrates dilated cortical veins without a nidus with a dural AVM (**Figs. 232 and 233**).

   (h) Mixed pial and dural AVMs—15 to 50% of pial AVMs have meningeal feeders.

5. Cavernous malformations

   (a) They are multilobulated berry–like structures full of blood of different ages. They are composed of closely approximated endothelial-lined sinusoidal spaces, large thin-walled vessels, no feeding artery, and **no intervening brain**. There are frequent calcifications and a surrounding **hemosiderin ring**. Eighty percent are supratentorial, but they may also be in the cerebellum, pons, and spinal cord. Ten percent are multiple and 5% are familial. The peak age of presentation is 20–40 years (**Fig. 234**).

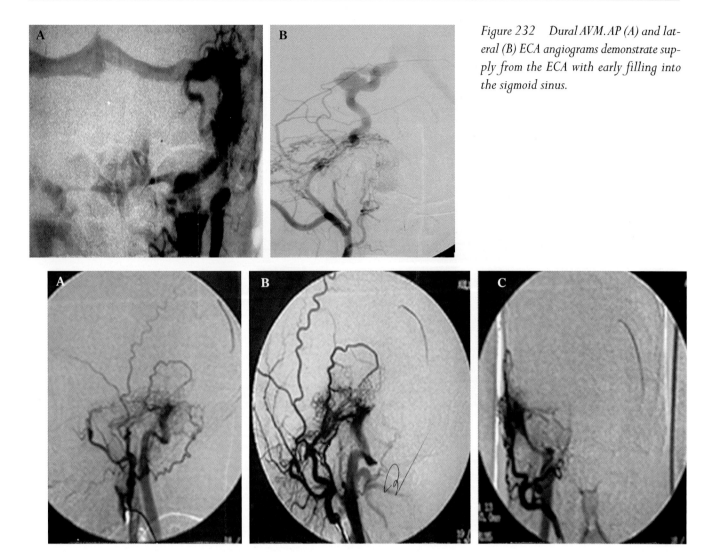

Figure 232   Dural AVM. AP (A) and lateral (B) ECA angiograms demonstrate supply from the ECA with early filling into the sigmoid sinus.

Figure 233   Dural AVM. Lateral (A), oblique (B), and AP (C) angiograms with filling of the sigmoid sinus through the ECA with a small dural nidus.

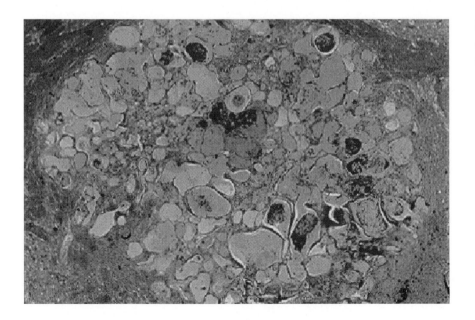

Figure 234   Cavernous malformation (H and E). Multiple thin-walled vessels without intervening brain tissue.

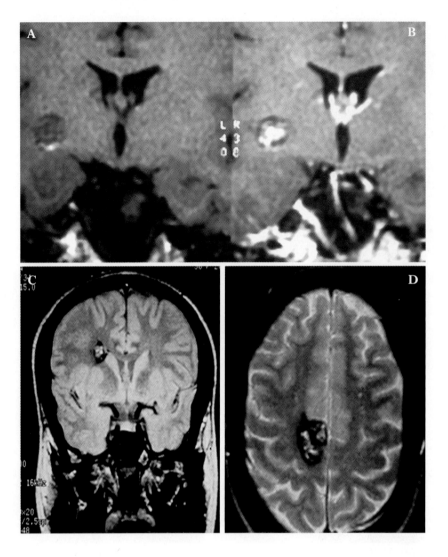

Figure 235   Cavernous malformation. Coronal T1-weighted MRIs noninfused (A) and infused (B), and coronal (C) and axial (D) T2-weighted MRIs demonstrating typical "popcorn" lesions with surrounding hemosiderin ring.

(b) CT may demonstrate the calcifications or a fluid-fluid level.

(c) The angiogram is normal and the MRI has a characteristic **"popcorn" lesion** that is hyperintense on T1-weighted MRI with a hypointense rim. They may or may not enhance (**Fig. 235**).

(d) Risk of hemorrhage is 0.5 to 1% per year, although it may be higher in the familial form in Hispanics.

6. Capillary telangiectasias—the second most common vascular malformation. They are small, multiple, clinically silent, firm capillary lesions, located in the white matter or classically the pons, and consist of multiple normal-sized and dilated thin vascular spaces without smooth muscle or elastic fibers. **There is usually normal brain between lesions.** Rarely there is evidence of old hemorrhage or gliosis. The angiogram is normal and the MRI reveals a lesion that is hypointense on T2-weighted images. In ROW syndrome, the mucocutaneous lesions are capillary telangiectasias, but the brain lesions are AVMs (**Fig. 236**).

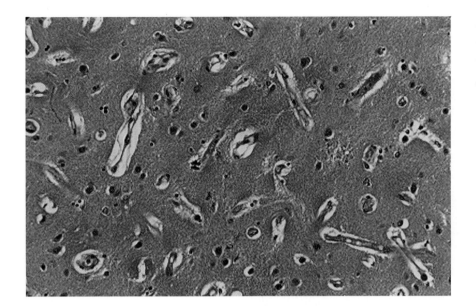

Figure 236   *Capillary telangiectasia (H and E). Multiple thin-walled vascular channels separated by normal brain parenchyma.*

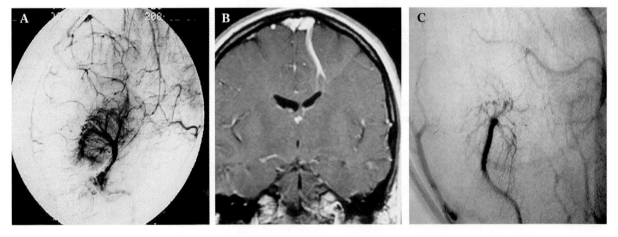

Figure 237   *Venous malformation. Angiograms (A and C) and infused MRI (B) demonstrating a "caput medusae" of small veins draining into a large irregular vein.*

7. Venous malformations—the most common vascular malformation. **There is intervening normal brain.** They consist of a large draining cortical vein receiving a collection of medullary veins (caput medusa) that usually occur near the angle of the ventricle. They rarely hemorrhage. They are caused by arrested development. Thirty-three percent are associated with cavernous malformations. They are usually solitary, although they are multiple with blue rubber nevus syndrome. They rarely require treatment (**Figs. 237 through 239**).

8. Venous varix—a single tortuous draining vein that is a normal variant. It is associated with AVMs.

9. Sinus pericranii—a large communication between intracranial and extracranial veins. It may be congenital or caused by trauma. It is a soft mass that changes with head position. It is associated with other malformations.

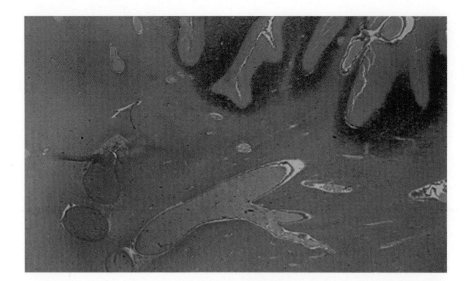

Figure 238   Venous malformation (H and E). Ectatic, large-diameter, thin-walled vessel.

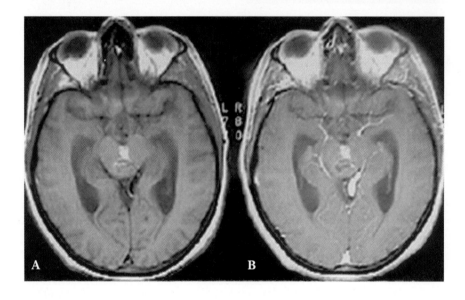

Figure 239   Cavernous malformations with associated venous malformation. Axial T1-weighted noninfused (A) and infused (B) MRIs demonstrating a posterior midbrain cavernous malformation draining into a venous malformation. Hemorrhage is present in the medial anterior midbrain.

XXI. CNS TRAUMA

A. Before the age of 44 years, trauma is the leading cause of death, and 50% of the deaths are from head trauma.

B. Abrasion—a scraping injury where a layer of tissue is removed.

C. Laceration—an injury creating a break in the tissues without tissue loss.

D. Contusion—a compressive injury to a tissue.

E. Ecchymosis—movement of blood from one extravascular site to another. Periorbital ecchymosis (racoon's eye) is into the upper and lower eyelids from an orbital roof fracture. Mastoid ecchymosis (Battle's sign) is from a petrous temporal fracture.

F. Concussion—a reversible transitory neurologic deficit associated with trauma and caused by rotational shear stress. There is loss of consciousness for < 24 hours by definition.

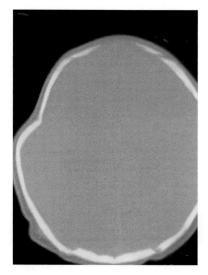

Figure 240   Ping-pong skull fracture. Axial CT with right-sided depressed fracture involving mainly the outer table.

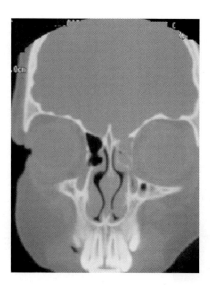

Figure 241   Cribriform plate skull fracture with CSF leak. Coronal CT bone window demonstrates left side cribriform plate fracture with opacification of the ethmoid sinus.

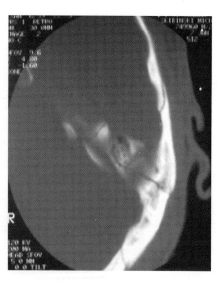

Figure 242   Longitudinal petrous bone fracture. Axial CT demonstrating fracture.

G. Fractures

1. Linear fracture—a line of fracture forms from the point of impact until the force is dissipated. Ten percent of adults with a linear skull fracture have a surgical lesion (mostly EDH). Linear fractures account for 75% of childhood skull fractures. Children < 3 years old have a risk of a **growing skull fracture** developing where a leptomeningeal cyst progressively protrudes through a dural tear.

2. Depressed fracture—caused by force to a more narrow surface area and has a higher frequency of parenchymal injury (**Fig. 240**).

3. Comminuted fracture—caused by a stronger force to a wider surface area.

4. Diastatic fracture—occurs when the fracture extends to and opens a suture. These are more common in childhood because the sutures are not as adherent.

5. Compound fracture—associated with open skin.

6. Basilar fracture—at the base of the skull. They may be linear, comminuted, or depressed (**Fig. 241 and 242**).

7. Nonaccidental fracture—suspect if multiple, depressed, width > 3 mm, growing fracture, more than one cranial bone involved, **nonparietal**, or with an associated injury.

H. Contusion

1. The second most common traumatic brain injury (after DAI) and has a lower occurrence of initial loss of consciousness.

2. Locations—temporal (50%), frontal (30%), and parasagittal/convexity (25%).

3. Definition—bruise of the cortical surface with hemorrhage from a torn vessel into the cortex. It affects the superficial layers unlike a stroke.

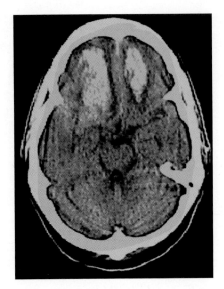

Figure 243   *Parenchymal contusion. Noninfused CT demonstrates bilateral frontal contusions.*

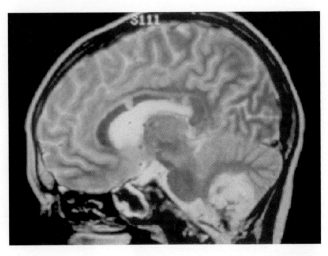

Figure 244   *Diffuse axonal injury. Sagittal T2-weighted MRI demonstrates high-intensity lesions of the corpus callosum.*

4. **Contre-coup** injury—caused by rotational shear. The anterior and middle skull bases have rigid sphenoid wings and petrous ridges. Rotation causes the **frontal and temporal cortices to sweep across** these structures and slow down, shearing the axons and vessels (**Fig. 243**).

5. **Coup** contusions—impact through the skull to the underlying brain. They occur at the **convexities**, are less common and less severe. The bones are usually intact.

6. It is less common to have contusions in children because they have a softer unmyelinated brain with smoother skull bases and more pliable skulls. Twenty percent of contusions develop delayed hemorrhages.

I. Diffuse axonal injury (DAI)—the most common traumatic brain injury (50%). There is immediate loss of consciousness. Petechiae are found in the **gray/white junction** (66%), **corpus callosum** (20%), dorsolateral rostral brain stem, and superior cerebellar peduncle. Axon retraction balls form first, followed by Wallerian degeneration. The injury may be due to shearing of axons but also to impaired transport and organelle accumulation with the axons separating after the edema resolves. DAI is best identified with MRI where it is hyperintense on T2-weighted MRI (**Fig. 244**).

J. Gunshot wounds—50% are associated with major vascular injuries. The wounding capacity depends on the energy of the missile. Low-velocity missiles travel at < 2000 ft/s (civilian bullets) and the damage is caused by the tract and a cavity four times the size of the bullet. High-velocity missiles travel at > 2000 ft/s (military bullets) and the cavity created is 30 times the size of the bullet because of high-energy shock waves.

K. Epidural hematoma (EDH)

1. They have a characteristic **lentiform biconvex shape, do not cross suture lines**, may cross dural attachments, and are most frequently in the temporoparietal region (**Fig. 245**).

2. They are seen in 3% of head injuries with peak age 10 to 30 years. They are rare before 2 years or after 60 years because at the extremes of age the dura is more adherent to the bone.

3. One third of EDHs have the characteristic lucid interval before deterioration. The hemorrhage is from the middle meningeal artery, a dural sinus, or a diploic vein.

4. Eighty-five percent are associated with a skull fracture, 43 to 75% with other brain lesions, and 13% with SDH. 5% are bilateral, and 5% are in the posterior fossa. Delayed formation occurs in 20% and delayed enlargement at 48 hours occurs in 20%.

5. The overall mortality is 5%, but it is less if the patient is awake on arrival.

L. Subdural hematoma (SDH)

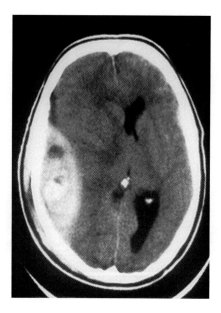

Figure 245   EDH. Noninfused CT demonstrates low-density unclotted hyperacute hemorrhage within the high-density biconvex (lentiform) clot.

1. They are **crescentic shaped, cross suture lines** but not dural attachments, and occur in 10 to 35% of severe head injuries. Fifty percent of patients present flaccid or decerebrate, and the mortality is 40 to 70%. Eight percent have a complete recovery (**Figs. 246 and 247**).

2. In one series, if surgery was performed before 6 hours, the mortality was 30% and after 6 hours it was 95%.

3. The hemorrhage is caused by tearing of a bridging vein by angular acceleration.

4. Fifty percent are associated with skull fractures. There is frequent SAH and DAI. 5% occur in the posterior fossa and 15% are bilateral.

5. Subacute SDH is 1 to 2 weeks old and chronic SDH is >3 weeks old.

6. Chronic SDH may rebleed (10 to 30%) because of stretching of bridging veins or by **neomembrane formation** over the calvarial surface's arachnoid with fibroblasts and fragile capillaries. The membranes enhance. Two percent of SDHs calcify.

7. Child abuse is associated with bilateral interhemispheric SDHs.

M. Subarachnoid hemorrhage (SAH)—the most common traumatic hemorrhage.

N. Intraventricular hemorrhage (IVH)—occurs in 1 to 5% of closed-head injuries and indicates severe trauma. It is also seen with hypertensive hemorrhages and ruptured AVMs.

O. Intraparenchymal hemorrhage (IPH)—associated with contusion or DAI.

P. Edema—there may be cytotoxic edema caused by brain injury and/or vasogenic edema caused by hyperemia with breakdown of the BBB. Vasogenic edema is seen in 15% of severe brain injuries and is more common in children.

Q. Vascular complications—aneurysm, pseudoaneurysm, dissection, laceration, and AVF (at the skull base, usually CCF, and may or may not be associated with a fracture).

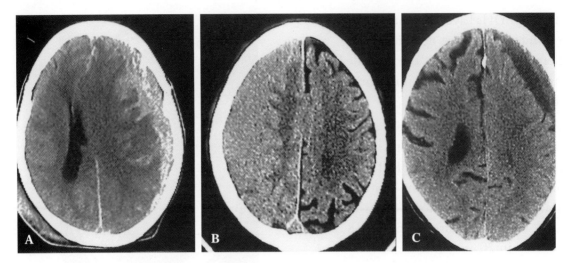

Figure 246   SDH. Noninfused CTs demonstrate (A) acute left SDH with concave (crescentic) high-density blood and associated SAH, (B) subacute right SDH with isodense blood, and (C) chronic left SDH with low-density blood.

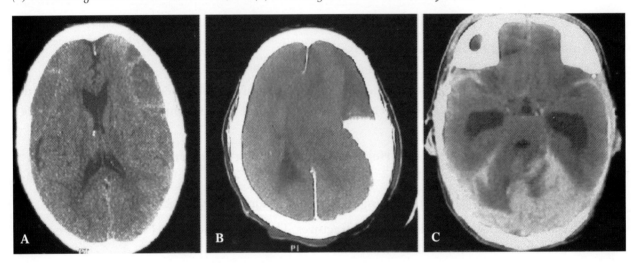

Figure 247   SDH. Noninfused CTs demonstrate (A) bilateral subacute SDH, (B) chronic left SDH with acute hemorrhage (fluid-fluid level), and (C) posterior fossa SDH.

R. Arterial dissections—associated with hypertension, migraines, activity, FMD, Marfan's disease, co-caine, OCPs, pharyngeal infections, syphilis, and trauma. The cervical ICA is affected by hyperextension and lateral flexion stretching the ICA over the transverse processes. Extracranial ICA dissections spare the carotid bulb and usually begin 2 cm distal to the bifurcation. Less commonly, intracranial dissections occur at the midsupraclinoid ICA where it is more mobile. Vertebral artery dissections occur between C2 and the skull.

S. Secondary complications of trauma

1. Increased ICP—the most common cause of death in trauma and is usually related to edema and/or hemorrhage.

2. Hypoxic injury—secondary to increased ICP, hypotension, hypoxia, or vasospasm (5 to 10% of cases), and usually occurs at the ACA/MCA territory junction, hippocampus, basal ganglia, and cerebellum.

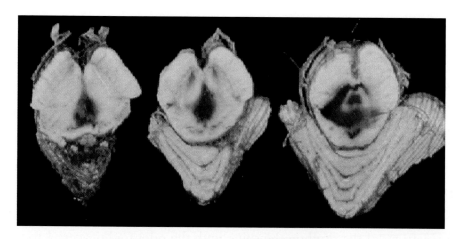

Figure 248   Duret hemorrhages (gross). Midbrain hemorrhages caused by herniation.

T. Sequelae of trauma—encephalomalacia, pneumocephalus, CSF leakage, cranial nerve palsies (especially the olfactory nerve), diabetes insipidus, cephalocele, leptomeningeal cyst, hydrocephalus, and long-term personality or cognitive changes (dementia).

U. Posttraumatic seizures—occur with 5% of closed-head injuries and 50% of penetrating injuries. Treat with 3 weeks of phenytoin (Dilantin) and then discontinue if no further seizures occur.

V. Postconcussive syndrome—characterized by headaches, lethargy, etc. in the weeks after a major head trauma.

W. Pediatric trauma—the infant's skull is malleable and thus tolerates much more deformity without a fracture developing. **Child abuse/nonaccidental trauma** is associated with multiple long bone fractures, chronic SDH, retinal hemorrhages, SDH of different ages, and multiple, complex, bilateral, and depressed skull fractures. Shaking an infant causes the hemispheres to rub along the falx, resulting in an **interhemispheric SDH**.

X. Diffuse cerebral swelling—occurs mainly in **children** after head trauma. It is caused by **hyperemia** with venous congestion, and manifests with severe swelling and ICP elevation.

Y. Herniation syndromes

1. Subfalcine herniation—the cingulate gyrus moves under the free edge of the falx and the ipsilateral foramen of Monro becomes trapped causing an ipsilateral large lateral ventricle and contralateral small lateral ventricle. The ACA may also be compressed.

2. Transtentorial herniation—usually a descending herniation with the uncus and parahippocampal gyrus being pushed over the tentorial edge. There is obliteration of the suprasellar cistern and inferomedial displacement of the anterior choroidal artery, PCOM, and PCA. The PCA may be compressed causing occipital strokes. The anterior choroidal artery and perforators may be compressed causing midbrain **Duret's hemorrhages** (these may also be caused by vessel stretching) and basal ganglia strokes. The contralateral brain stem is compressed against **Kernohan's notch** producing ipsilateral hemiparesis (false localizing sign). Ascending transtentorial herniation causes effacement of the superior vermian cistern, quadrigeminal cistern, and fourth ventricle (**Fig. 248**).

3. Transalar (transphenoidal) herniation—the frontal lobe may descend against the greater sphenoid wing or the temporal lobe may ascend against it.

4. Tonsillar herniation—the cerebellar tonsils descend through the foramen magnum.

XXII. SKULL DISEASES

A. Fibrous dysplasia—presents in young adulthood. It may be either monostotic (70% of cases and 25% involve the skull/face) or polyostotic (30% of cases and 50% involve the skull/face). It expands and replaces normal bony medullary spaces with vascular fibrocellular tissue. CT demonstrates thickened sclerotic bone with **"ground-glass" expanded diploe**. It is hypointense on T1-weighted images and enhances. There may be sclerotic orbits and skull bases causing lionlike facies. Albright's syndrome is unilateral polyostotic disease and precocious puberty (see Figs. 158 through 160).

B. Paget's disease—may be monostotic or polyostotic. Early in the course, it causes destruction and late it causes sclerosis. There is bony expansion that may cause basilar invagination.

C. Basilar impression/invagination—settling of the skull on the spine with the odontoid process 4 to 5 mm above McGregor's line or occipital condyles above the plane of the foramen magnum. Evaluation includes **McRae's line** (foramen magnum diameter 35 mm $\pm$4), **Chamberlin's line** (diagonal line from the hard palate to the posterior foramen magnum, the odontoid should not have $\frac{1}{3}$ of its length above it), and **McGregor's line** (line from the hard palate to the most caudal portion of the occipital curve, odontoid tip should be <4 mm above the line). Symptoms include lower cranial nerve palsies, headache, and limb spasticity. It is associated with atlantoaxial fusion, osteogenesis imperfecta, rheumatoid arthritis, and Paget's disease.

D. Platybasia—flattened skull base with an increased angle of the clivus to the spine or clivus to the anterior fossa >135 degrees. It is associated with basilar invagination or Chiari I malformation.

E. Wormian bones—small intrasutural bones, usually in the lambdoid suture. They are seen with cleidocranial dysostosis, cretinism, osteogenesis imperfecta, chronic hydrocephalus, and as a normal variant.

F. Hemangioma—may involve the frontal or parietal skull, and has a **honeycomb pattern** with radiating spicules. See section XXIV B.

G. Foramen magnum lesions—may classically cause weakness of first the ipsilateral UE, followed by the ipsilateral LE, the contralateral LE, and then the contralateral UE.

H. Also see Section IX.

XXIII. DEVELOPMENTAL SPINAL LESIONS

A. Spinal lipoma

    1. It is associated with occult spinal lesions and the most common cause of tethered cord.

    2. Lipomyelomeningocele—accounts for 84% of spinal lipomas and 20% of skin covered masses. It has a female predominance. Symptoms include bladder dysfunction, decreased sensation, and orthopedic deformities. It is not associated with Chiari II malformations (**Figs. 249 and 250**).

    3. Filum terminale fibrolipoma—accounts for 12% of spinal lipomas and is formed by faulty retrogressive differentiation. It is frequently asymptomatic.

    4. Intradural lipoma—accounts for 4% of spinal lipomas. It occurs most commonly in the cervical and thoracic spines and the spinal cord is open posteriorly (**Figs. 251 and 252**).

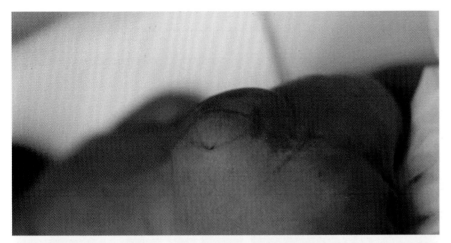

Figure 249   Lipomyelomeningocele. Skin-covered lumbar hump.

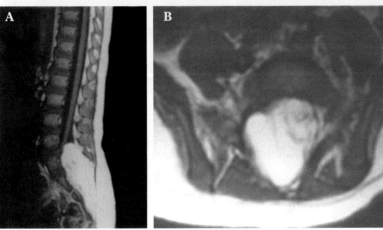

Figure 250   Lipomyelomeningocele. Sagittal (A) and axial (B) T1-weighted noninfused MRIs demonstrating the spinal cord terminating in a dorsal lipoma that extends to the sacral surface.

B. Tethered cord—when not associated with a lipoma, it may be caused by a **thick filum terminale** preventing the spinal cord from ascending in the spinal canal. The low-lying conus and a filum > 1.5 mm in diameter is identified on MRI or CT. Tethered cord is also associated with a spinal lipoma (72%). It most commonly presents at 3 to 35 years with no sex predominance. Symptoms include spasticity, pain, decreased sensation, bladder dysfunction, and kyphoscoliosis (25%) (**Fig. 253**).

C. Caudal spinal anomalies (malformations associated with GI or GU abnormalities)

1. Caudal regression syndrome—consists of lumbosacral agenesis, imperforate anus, genital malformations, renal dysplasia, and sirenomelia (fused legs). It may be mild or severe (**Fig. 254**).

2. Terminal myelocystocele—consists of posterior spina bifida or partial sacral agenesis with tethered cord and hydromyelia.

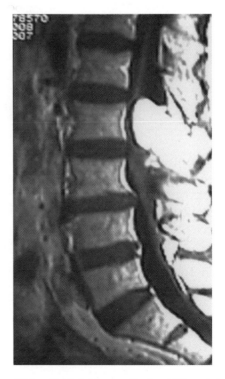

Figure 251   Spinal lipoma. Sagittal T1-weighted MRI demonstrates a high-intensity lipoma extending from the subcutaneous tissue to the spinal cord.

185

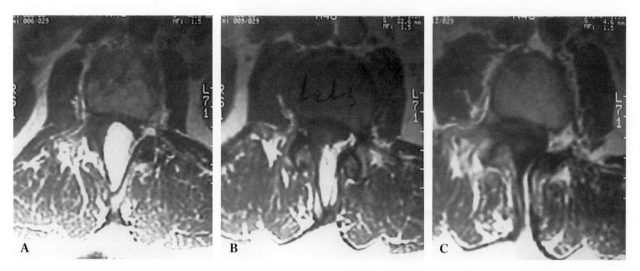

Figure 252   Spinal lipoma. Axial T1-weighted MRIs (A to C) demonstrating a lipoma extending through a bifid spine to the middle of the spinal cord.

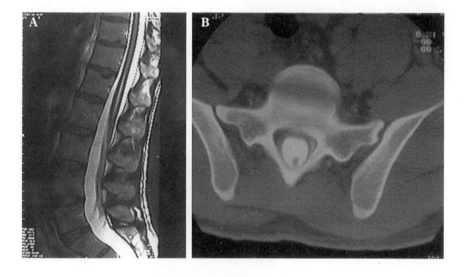

Figure 253   Tethered cord. T2-weighted sagittal MRI (A) and axial CT myelogram (B) demonstrate the conus extending to L3 with a small terminal syrinx and a thickened filum terminale.

3. Anterior sacral meningocele—extends into the pelvis by an anterior defect. It may be a form of caudal regression syndrome and is associated with NF1 and Marfan's syndrome.

4. Occult intrasacral meningocele—the arachnoid herniates through a sacral dural defect.

5. Sacrococcygeal teratoma—the most common pre-sacral mass in children.

D. Split notocord syndrome—a persistent connection exists between the gut and the dorsal ectoderm. It may be caused by an adhesion between the endoderm and ectoderm.

E. Diastematomyelia—split cord with a fibrous, bony (50%), or cartilaginous septum. It is a local split with a complete cord above and below. Fifty percent have a single dural tube; 85% have vertebral body anomalies, 40% have thick filums, 50 to 75% have **cutaneous stigmata** (hair patch, nevi, lipoma, etc.), 50% have orthopedic problems (i.e., club foot), and 90% have nonspecific neurologic symptoms (pain, weakness, and bladder dysfunction). It is most common in the **lumbar area** (T9-S1 85%). Twenty percent of Chiari II malformations have an associated diastematomyelia. There is a female predominance **(Fig. 255)**.

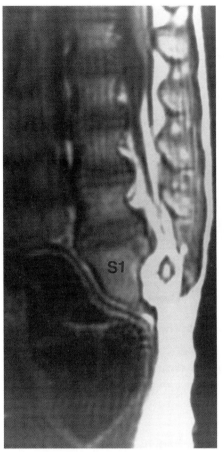

Figure 254   Sacral agenesis. Sagittal T1-weighted MRI demonstrates agenesis of the sacrum below S1 with an associated lipoma

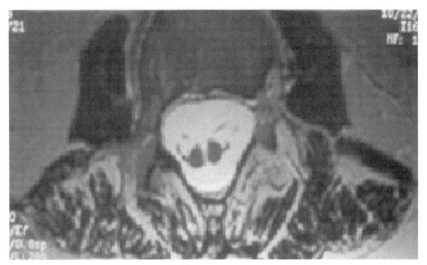

Figure 255   Diastematomyelia. Axial T2-weighted MRI demonstrates the dual spinal cords.

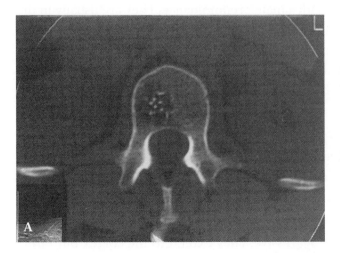

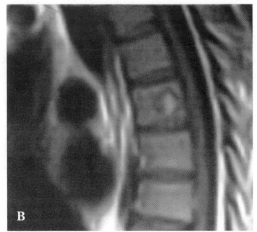

Figure 256   (A)Vertebral hemangioma. Axial CT demonstrating "polka dot" lesion in the vertebral body. (B) T2-weighted MRI of the thoracic spine demonstrating the hemangioma.

F. Enterogenous cyst—caused by failure of the notochord and foregut to separate. They are thin-walled fluid-filled masses lined by columnar/cuboidal cells with some goblet cells. Peak age is 0 to 20 years with a male predominance. They usually form in the midline, are intradural extramedullary, and are most commonly in the thoracic spine (42%) and cervical spine (32%). Symptoms include pain, myelopathy, and septic or chemical meningitis. Forty-three percent have associated vertebral anomolies.

G. Hydromyelia—a fluid collection within the spinal cord **lined by ependymal cells**, and thus a dilation of the central canal. This contrasts with a syrinx cavity that is not lined by ependymal cells. Twenty percent communicate with the fourth ventricle by way of the obex, and these are associated with hydrocephalus, SAH, meningitis, and cancer. Eighty percent are noncommunicating and are associated with Chiari I and II malformations, trauma, tumor, and cord compression. Symptoms are a **capelike loss of pain and temperature**, pain ($<$50%), and UMN findings in the LEs with lower motor findings in the UEs (80%) (see Fig. 11).

XXIV. SPINAL TUMORS

A. General—the spinal bone marrow contains more of the red marrow than the yellow variety before age 7 years and thus enhances. The DRG have less of a BBB and also may enhance. Spinal canal tumors may be intramedullary (5%, ependymoma and astrocytoma), intradural-extramedullary (40%, meningioma at any location or schwannoma mostly in the thoracic spine), or epidural (55%, metastatic).

B. Bone tumors

1. Hemangioma—peak age 30 to 50 years, female predominance, benign, and found in 10% of autopsies. Seventy-five percent are spinal (lower thoracic and lumbar) and they are usually in the **vertebral body** and rarely in the posterior elements (10%). One percent are extraosseous and 30% are multiple. CT demonstrates the **"polka dot" lesion** in the vertebral body. They may be vascular, fatty, and enhancing. Most are asymptomatic (60%), although they can expand and fracture the vertebral body causing cord compression. Symptoms include pain (20%) and neurologic deficit (20%, mainly after hemorrhage) (**Fig. 256**).

2. Osteoid osteoma—peak age 10 to 20 years with a male predominance. They are usually in the long bones of the lower limb and the spine is involved in 10% (**lumbar neural arch**, rarely the body). The CT reveals dense sclerosis around a lytic lesion with a central calcified **nidus of osteoid** and woven bone. They are usually $<$2 cm and if they are larger, they are likely to be osteoblastoma. They account for 6% of benign spinal tumors. Symptoms include scoliosis and pain that responds to ASA (**Fig. 257**).

3. Osteoblastoma (giant osteoid osteoma)—$>$**2 cm** in size rare, peak age 20 years, and have a male predominance. They occur in the **posterior elements** of the cervical spine and cause pain. Ten percent recur and they may grow aggressively.

4. Giant cell tumor—peak age 10 to 40 years with a female predominance. They are mainly in the ends of long bones and occasionally in the **sacral body** but rarely elsewhere in the spine. They are benign, lytic, expansile, and locally aggressive. They extend to the cortex but rarely beyond. They frequently hemorrhage and rarely calcify. Symptoms include pain and neurologic deficits. They recur frequently and 10% undergo malignant change.

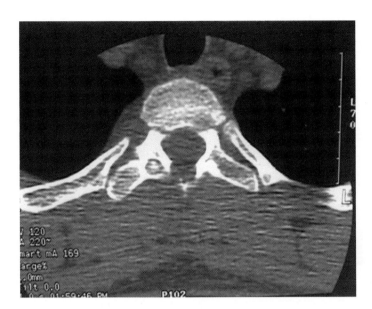

Figure 257   Osteoid osteoma. Axial CT demonstrating lytic lesion with surrounding sclerosis and a central nidus in the right laminar base.

5. Osteochondroma—peak age 20 years with a male predominance. Four percent are spinal and usually are on the **C2 spinous process or transverse processes at other levels**. They are multiple in 12%. They arise from lateral displacement of the epiphyseal growth cartilage and have a bony projection with a medullary cavity contiguous with the parent bone and covered with cartilage.

6. Aneurysmal bone cyst

   (a) Usually present before 20 years and have a female predominance.

   (b) They usually occur at the metaphyses of long bones but 20% are spinal, usually in the cervical and thoracic **posterior elements**. They are nonneoplastic and of unknown cause. They may begin as a hemorrhage into some other type of lesion.

   (c) They are multiloculated, **expansile**, **lytic**, vascular, and surrounded by **eggshell cortical bone** and no calcifications.

   (d) Microscopic examination reveals thin-walled blood cavities without endothelium or elastic lamina and frequent multinucleated giant cells.

   (e) Symptoms include pain, swelling, fracture, and compression.

   (f) They frequently recur and are associated with chondroblastoma, giant cell tumor, osteoblastoma, and fibrous dysplasia (**Fig. 258**).

7. Eosinophilic granuloma—peak age 5 to 10 years, benign, nonneoplastic, and in the Langerhan's cell histiocytosis group (see Chapter 4 section VII R for more information). They are **lytic without surrounding sclerosis** and are a classic cause of a single collapsed vertebral body. They enhance and are hyperintense on T2-weighted MRI (see Fig. 156).

8. Chordoma—peak age 50 to 60 years with male predominance. Located at the ends of the spinal axis: **sacral** (50%), **clivus** (35%), and less often in the vertebral bodies (15%). They

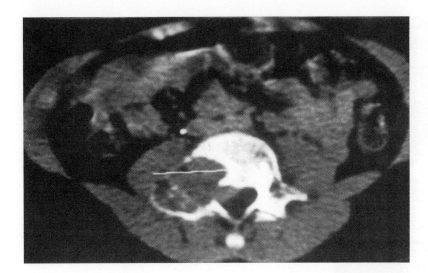

Figure 258   Aneurysmal bone cyst. Non-infused axial CT demonstrates expansive lytic lesion surrounded by a thin rim of cortical bone.

are lytic soft tissue masses with vacuolated **physaliphorous cells** with mucin. They may contain calcifications (30 to 70%). Chordomas are derived from **notochord remnants** and are the most common primary sacral tumors. See section VIII O for more detail.

9. Lymphoma—peak age is 40 to 65 years with a male predominance. Usually non-Hodgkin's lymphoma. Median survival is 2 years. Treatment is with chemotherapy and radiation.

10. Ewing's sarcoma—peak age is 10 to 20 years with a male predominance. They are usually non-spinal and only involve the spine by metastasis.

11. Osteosarcoma—peak age 10 to 25 years with a male predominance. It is rarely spinal and is more common with Paget's disease or radiation. CT reveals matrix calcifications with a sunburst pattern.

12. Chondrosarcoma—peak age 50 to 70 years with a male predominance. They may arise from a solitary osteochondroma (1%) or multiple exostoses (20%).

13. Fibrosarcomas—rare.

14. Plasmacytoma—a solitary lesion of plasma cells (called multiple myeloma when multiple). Peak age is 50 years and the **vertebral body** is the most common location. It is lytic.

C. Epidural lesions (The most common lesions are degenerative, traumatic, or metastatic tumors)

1. Metastatic tumors—most frequently breast, lung, and prostate. In children, the most common are Ewing's sarcoma and neuroblastoma. They are usually in the lower thoracic and lumbar spine, correlating with areas having the highest concentration of red marrow. Most are lytic except breast and prostate, which are sclerotic and blastic. They usually enter the spinal canal by way of the neural foramina and cause circumferential compression. Do not perform a lumbar puncture below the obstruction (**Figs. 259 and 260**).

2. Epidural lipomatosis—fat accumulation in the epidural space with male predominance. It usually develops in the thoracic or lumbar spine and presents with pain and weakness, is associated

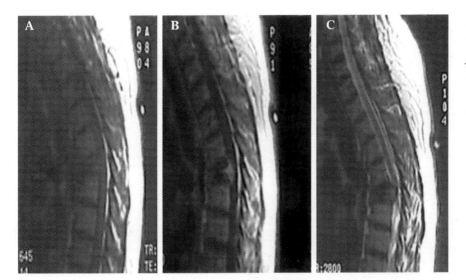

Figure 259   Epidural/vertebral metasta-tic tumor. Sagittal noninfused (A) and in-fused (B) T1-weighted, and T2-weighted (C) MRIs demonstrating enhancing thoracic ver-tebral body lesion with extension into ven-tral epidural space.

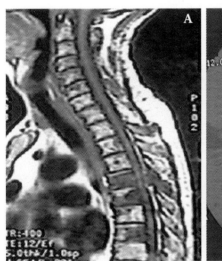
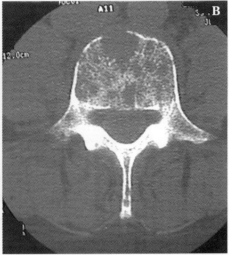

Figure 260   Multiple myeloma. Sagit-tal infused T1-weighted MRI (A) and axial CT (B) demonstrating diffuse bony involvement.

with obesity and steroid use. Treatment is by weight loss, discontinuation of steroids if being used, and decompressive surgery if necessary (**Fig. 261**).

3. Spinal angiolipoma—rare, peak age < 10 years, female predominance, and is usually in the dorsal epidural thoracic spine.

4. Extradural arachnoid cyst—usually thoracic, protrudes through a dural defect and may cause cord compression.

D. Intradural/extramedullary lesions

1. Nerve sheath tumors—the most common spinal tumors (30%). Schwannomas are more com-mon than neurofibromas (unencapsulated, no cystic or hemorrhagic degeneration, nerves run through them, and fusiform-shaped). Forty percent of patients with nerve sheath tumors have NF. Locations are intradural/extramedullary (70%), extradural (15%), dumbbell (15%), and

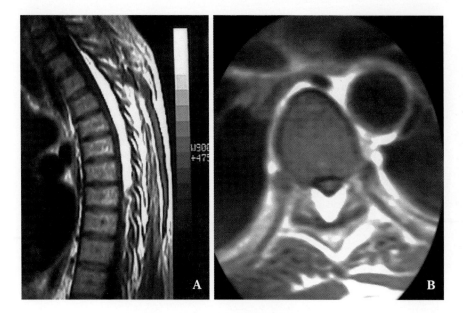

Figure 261   *Epidural lipomatosis. Sagittal (A) and axial (B) T1-weighted MRIs demonstrating dorsal high-intensity adipose tissue accumulation with cord compression.*

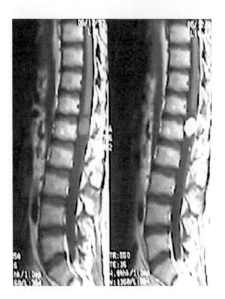

Figure 262   *Intradural extramedullary schwannoma. Sagittal noninfused (A) and infused (B) T1-weighted MRIs demonstrating a T12/L1 circumscribed enhancing lesion.*

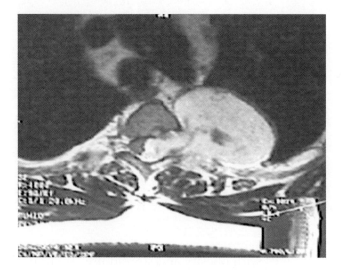

Figure 263   *Intradural extramedullary dumbbell neurofibroma. Infused axial T1-weighted MRI demonstrating a large circumscribed enhancing tumor extending through the widened left intervertebral foramen.*

intramedullary (1%). Symptoms include pain, radiculopathy, and myelopathy. See Chapter 4 section VIII T for more information (**Figs. 262 and 263**).

2. Meningioma—accounts for 25% of spinal tumors, peak age is 40 to 60 years, and has a female predominance. It is usually in the **thoracic spine**, is occasionally multiple, and is intradural (90%), extradural (5%), and dumbbell (5%). Symptoms are motor and sensory deficits. Less than 10% recur. There are rarely bone erosions or calcifications (**Fig. 264**).

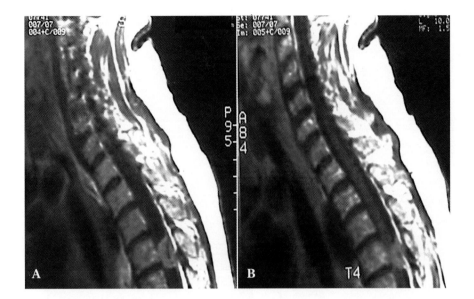

Figure 264   Intradural extramedullary meningioma. T1-weighted noninfused MRIs (A and B) with dorsal lesion extending along dural base.

3. Paraganglioma—rare, usually in the cauda equina, from accessory organs of the PNS (carotid body, glomus jugulare, para-aortic, mediastinal, and pheochromocytoma), encapsulated, hemorrhagic, and enhancing.

4. Epidermoid—may be congenital or acquired.

5. Dermoid—congenital, accounts for 20% of intradural masses < 1 year, 50% are intramedullary and 50% are extramedullary.

6. Neurenteric cyst—**ventral** to the thoracic spinal cord.

7. Arachnoid cyst—usually dorsal to the thoracic spinal cord.

8. Hypertrophic neuropathies—dejerrine-Sottas and Charcot-Marie-Tooth diseases. There may be intradural and extradural onion bulb formations.

9. Metastatic tumors—GBM, anaplastic astrocytoma, ependymoma, medulloblastoma, pineal tumors, germinoma, choroid plexus papilloma, lung carcinoma, breast carcinoma, melanoma, lymphoma, and leukemia. These have an 80% mortality in 4 months.

E. Intramedullary tumors

1. Ependymoma

(a) They account for 60% of intramedullary tumors and are the **most common intramedullary tumor in adults**.

(b) Cellular type—usually **cervical**, peak age 43 years, female predominance, circumscribed, frequently cystic or hemorrhagic, and causes symmetric cord expansion and pain (**Fig. 265**).

(c) Myxopapillary type—occurs at the **conus** or **filum**, peak age 28 years, male predominance, slow growing, may metastasize to the lymph nodes, bone, or lung, and 20% destroy bone (**Fig. 266**).

(d) They are isointense on T1-weighted images, hyperintense on T2-weighted images, and enhancing.

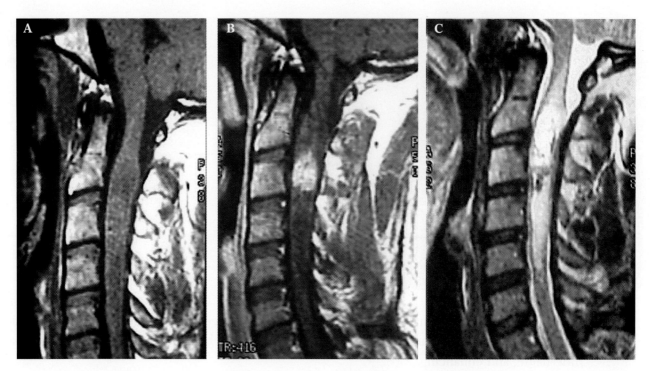

Figure 265   Intramedullary ependymoma. Sagittal T1-weighted noninfused (A) and infused (B) and T2-weighted (C) MRIs demonstrating enhancing expansile lesion in the central cervical spinal cord.

2. Astrocytoma—accounts for 30% of intramedullary tumors and is the **most common intramedullary tumor in children**. They are usually **cervical**, peak age 21 years, no sex predominance, low grade (75% in adults and 90% in children), frequently cause an eccentric cyst and syrinx, and are of the fibrillary type. They can cause scoliosis. Cervical astrocytomas usually enhance on CT and MRI (**Figs. 267 and 268**).

3. Hemangioblastoma—accounts for 5% of intramedullary tumors, peak age is 30 years, 50% are thoracic, and 40% are cervical. Seventy-five percent are intramedullary and 15% are intradural/extramedullary. Twenty percent are multiple. Thirty percent are associated with VHL. They are usually cystic with a vascular nodule and have dilated feeding vessels on angiography (see Figs. 178 and 179).

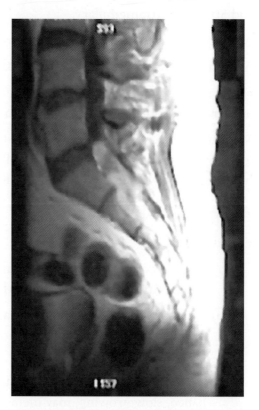

Figure 266   Myxopapillary ependymoma. Sagittal infused T1-weighted MRI demonstrates enhancing nodular mass filling the distal spinal canal.

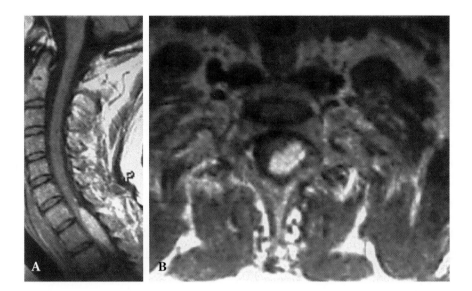

Figure 267   Intramedullary astrocytoma. Sagittal (A) and axial (B) infused T1-weighted MRIs demonstrating left-sided eccentric cervical mass.

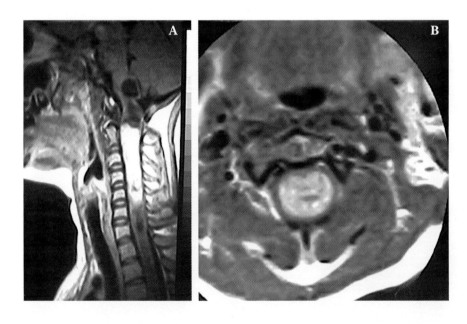

Figure 268   Intramedullary juvenile pilocytic astrocytoma. Sagittal (A) and axial (B) infused T1-weighted MRIs demonstrate the enhancing tumor with the associated syrinx extending into the brain stem.

4. Others—rarely there are oligodendrocytes, ganglioglioma, schwannomas, and metastases.

5. The most common symptom of intramedullary tumors is pain.

XXV. SPINAL VASCULAR DISEASES

A. Intramedullary hemorrhages—usually due to a vascular malformation, tumor, trauma, or anticoagulation.

B. Aneurysms—peak age 20 years with no sex predominance. Seventy percent are on the anterior spinal artery, usually cervical or thoracic. They are usually associated with AVMs' feeding arteries and do not occur at branch points. Presentation is SAH (85%) and neural compression (15%).

C. Spinal AVMs (an AVM has a true nidus and an AVF does not)

1. Type 1—the most frequent spinal arteriovenous malformation (AVM) (actually a **dural AVF**). Peak age is 40 to 70 years with a male predominance. It usually occurs in the dorsal lower thoracic spine or near the conus. It is usually **acquired**. There is a single transdural arterial feeder that goes to an intradural arterialized vein over multiple segments. There is rostral venous drainage. The nidus is in or adjacent to the dura around a nerve root. Symptoms are progressive neurologic deterioration caused by **venous hypertension**. It has **low pressure but high flow**. It is **less likely to hemorrhage** and is not associated with aneurysms. A good surgical outcome is obtained in 88% (**Fig. 269**).

2. Type 2 (**glomus AVM**)—**intramedullary**, has multiple feeders, drains into a venous plexus around the cord, usually dorsal cervicomedullary, affects younger people, and is **congenital**. It presents acutely with **hemorrhage** and has both **high flow and high pressure**.

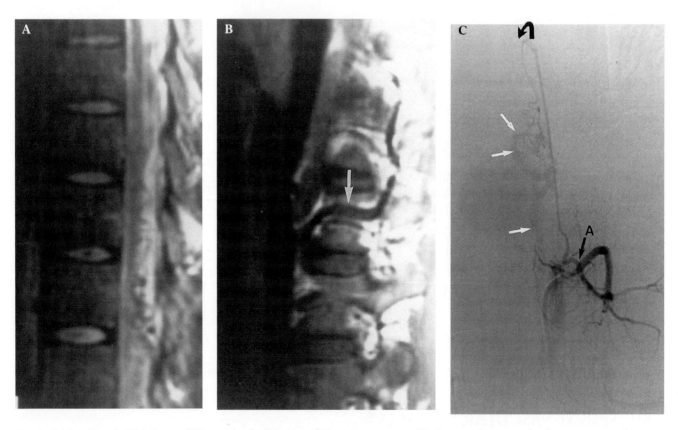

Figure 269   Spinal AVM. Sagittal T2-weighted MRIs (A and B) and angiogram (C) demonstrate upper lumbar segment with vascular blush and enlarged draining veins.

3. Type 3 (**juvenile AVM**)—rare, large, **intramedullary and extramedullary malformation** with **multiple extraspinal feeders**. It has **high pressure and high flow**, more frequent **hemorrhage** and vascular steal symptoms, and is associated with arterial and venous aneurysms. It has bidirectional venous drainage. It involves the entire cross-section of the cord. A good surgical outcome is obtained in 49% of cases.

4. Type 4—**intradural/extramedullary AVF**, anterior to the spinal cord, fed by the anterior spinal artery, usually near the conus and peak age is 20 to 50 years. It has **low pressure but high flow**, **rarely hemorrhages**, and symptoms are progressive by **venous congestion**.

5. **Foix-Alajouanine syndrome**—subacute necrotizing myelitis, especially in the gray matter, usually with a type 1 AVM, and caused by venous hypertension.

6. Klippel-Trénaunay-Weber syndrome—a spinal cord AVM with a cutaneous vascular nevus and an enlarged finger or arm (if cervical).

D. Cavernous malformations—rare, peak age 20 to 50 years, female predominance, usually thoracic, occasionally multiple, may hemorrhage, and angiogram is usually normal (**Fig. 270**).

E. Venous malformations—rare.

F. Capillary telangiectasias—rarely identified during life, but frequently found at autopsy.

G. Spinal cord stroke

1. It usually occurs in patients with severe atherosclerosis, may be caused by hypotension, commonly affects the midthoracic portion, involves the ventral posterior horns and the dorsolateral anterior horns, and has relative white matter sparing.

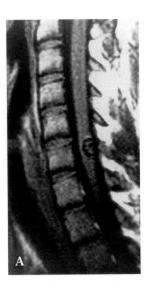 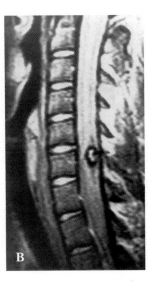

Figure 270   Spinal cord cavernous malformation. Sagittal T1-(A) and T2-weighted (B) MRIs demonstrating the lesion with surrounding hemosiderin ring within the cervical spinal cord.

2. Watershed areas—anterior/posterior spinal arteries, central/peripheral blood supply, and at the upper/middle/lower segments. An aortic branch injury may reduce the thoracic blood supply.

3. Etiologies—cross-clamping the aorta > 18 minutes, syphilis, atherosclerosis, embolism, aortic dissection, and spondylosis (usually affects the ASA and preserves the posterior columns). Very rarely there may be a fibrocartilage embolus from a disc to a vessel.

4. Venous thrombosis—may cause hemorrhage and may have sudden or slow onset of neurologic deficit.

5. Anterior spinal artery syndrome—from similar causes as the preceding. It is characterized by weakness and dissociated sensory loss (loss of spinothalamic pain and temperature sensation with sparing of posterior column function).

H. Decompression sickness (caisson disease)—intravascular accumulation of N_2 with vessel obstruction. It frequently causes spinal cord dysfunction in the posterior columns of the thoracic cord.

XXVI. SPINAL INFECTIONS

A. Pyogenic osteomyelitis

1. It is usually caused by **_Staphylococcus aureus_** (60%), and _Enterobacter_ (30%).

2. The infection reaches the spine by (1) hematogenous spread (the most common route, comes from the skin, GU system, lungs, or Batson's venous plexus), (2) contiguous spread, and (3) iatrogenic transmission.

3. In adults, the infection begins in the subchondral body and spreads to the disc space.

4. In children, the infection starts in the vascular disc space.

5. Peak age is 50 to 60 years with a male predominance.

6. The lumbar spine is affected most frequently followed by the thoracic spine.

7. Symptoms are pain, with or without fever, increased ESR, and leukocytosis.

8. X-ray is usually normal for 10 days and then demonstrates **end-plate erosion and disc space narrowing**. MRI is hypointense on T1-weighted images, hyperintense on T2-weighted images, and enhancing (**Figs. 271 and 272**).

9. Risk factors include IVDA and immunocompromised states.

B. Granulomatous osteomyelitis—caused by TB and fungus. The spine is involved in 6% of TB cases (Pott's disease). Peak age is 40 years with no sex predominance. It affects the lower thoracic and upper lumbar spine. Ninety percent of cases involve at least two bodies and 50% at least three bodies. Skip lesions are common. Fifty-five to 95% have an associated paraspinal abscess. There is slow progression of the disease with wedging and gibbus formation. Most cases eventually fuse. The risk increases with debilitation, immunosuppression, alcoholism, and IVDA.

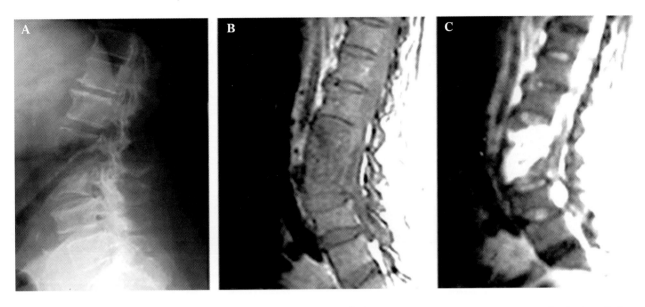

Figure 271   Osteomyelitis. Lateral x-ray film (A) demonstrating L2/3 end-plate erosion and sagittal T1-weighted (B) and T2-weighted (C) MRIs demonstrating the vertebral body signal changes extending across the L2/3 disc space.

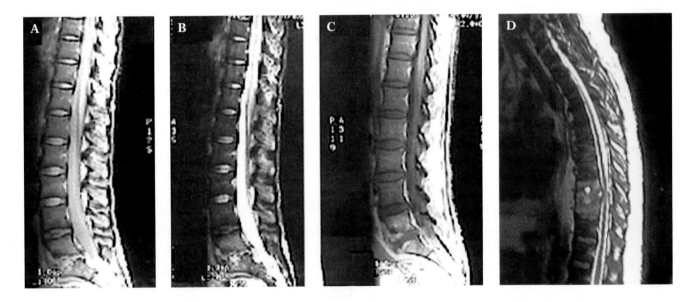

Figure 272   Discitis. Proton density (A), T2-weighted (B), and infused T1-weighted (C) MRIs demonstrating the L5/S1 enhancing disc inflammation. (D) T2-weighted MRI of the thoracic spine demonstrating Pott's disease with diskitis and osteomyelitis at T7 and 8.

C. Epidural abscess—usually caused by ***Staphylococcus aureus*** and peak age is 50 years with a male predominance. The infection is caused by bacterial seeding from the skin, lung, or bladder. It is associated with osteomyelitis and discitis (80%) and is frequently multilevel. Symptoms include fever, pain, and neurologic deficit. Initially, a phlegmon forms followed by liquid pus. The risk increases with diabetes mellitus, IVDA, and trauma. Symptoms may be due to direct neural compression or ischemia from venous compression or thrombosis (**Fig. 273**).

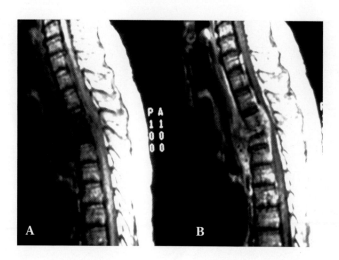

Figure 273   Spinal epidural abscess. Sagittal T1-weighted noninfused (A) and infused (B) MRIs demonstrating thoracic osteomyelitis with a ventral enhancing epidural abscess.

D. Subdural abscess—rare.

E. Abscess—rare.

F. Meningitis and myelitis—see Chapter 4 section VI.

XXVII. SPINAL INFLAMMATORY DISEASES

A. Acute transverse myelitis—affects all ages, no sex predominance, usually thoracic, and causes de-myelination. The MRI is normal in 50% of patients in the acute stage. It is associated with acute in-fection, post-infection, post-vaccination, autoimmune diseases, SLE, MS, and malignancies. The prognosis is variable and there are frequently permanent deficits.

B. Necrotizing myelopathy

    1. Devic's disease (neuromyelitis optica)—progressive fulminant demyelination of the optic nerve and spinal cord. It can result in blindness and paraplegia. It is associated with MS, varicella-zoster, mumps, rubeola, mononucleosis, TB, SLE, and tetanus booster. It tends to be more severe and monophasic than MS. See Chapter 4 section XVI for more information (**Fig. 274**).

    2. Lupus myelitis—usually at or below the thoracic level and has a variable course.

    3. Paraneoplastic necrotizing myelopathy—usually with lung or lymphoreticular cancers, suba-cute or rapid progression, and absence of inflammatory cells.

    4. Idiopathic.

C. Radiation myelopathy

    1. Usually a chronic progressive myelopathy and most frequently occurs after radiation for na-sopharyngeal carcinoma in the cervical spine.

    2. Symptoms usually occur 12 to 15 months after radiation and include **painless paresthesias** and dysesthesias, with sensory loss more common than motor loss.

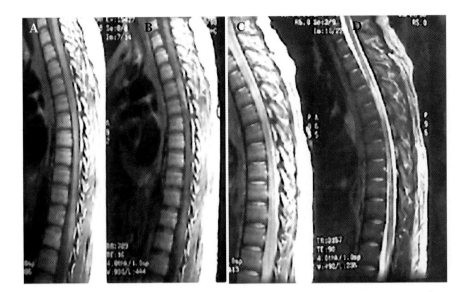

Figure 274   Devic's disease. Sagittal noninfused (A) and infused (B) T1-weighted, proton density (C), and T2-weighted (D) MRIs demonstrating upper thoracic inflammation extending over three levels.

3. Pathologic examination demonstrates coagulative necrosis affecting the white matter more than the gray matter and thrombosed hyalinized vessels (**Fig. 275**).

4. Postradiation changes to the vertebral bodies include hyperintensity on T1-weighted images due to increased fat content in the marrow (**Fig. 47**).

5. Treatment is with steroids.

6. The risk is decreased by keeping the total radiation dose < 6000 rad, the weekly dose < 900 rad, and the daily dose < 200 rad.

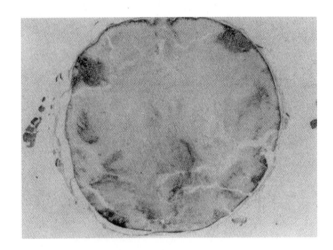

Figure 275   Radiation myelopathy. Coagulation necrosis.

D. Amyotropic lateral sclerosis (ALS)—see Chapter 4, section XV.

E. Postpolio syndrome—decompensation of surviving muscle without reserve. There is no further inflammation.

F. Anterior horn diseases—poliomyelitis, ALS, CJD, Werdnig-Hoffmann disease, and Kugelberg-Welander syndrome.

G. Myelopathy differential diagnosis—congenital degeneration (Freidrich's ataxia), radiation, AIDS, viral, compression, vascular malformation, toxic (ETOH), and metabolic (B$_{12}$) (**Figs. 276 through 282**).

H. Vertebral inflammatory diseases

1. Ankylosing spondylitis—presents at 10 to 30 years and affects 1.4% of the population at a site where a ligament attaches to a bone. It is an autoimmune disease causing sacroiliac and lumbar

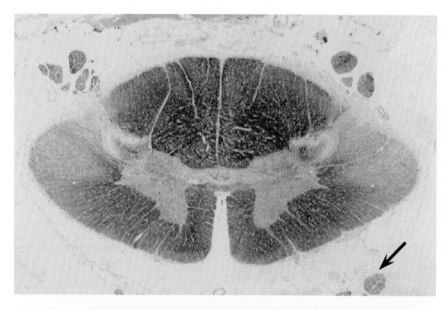

Figure 276   Amyotropic lateral sclerosis (ALS) (LFB). Degeneration of the lateral corticospinal tracts with atrophic demyelinated ventral roots (arrow) compared with the dorsal roots.

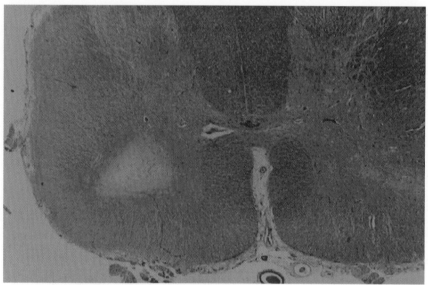

Figure 277   Poliomyelitis (H and E). Cystic degeneration of the anterior horn.

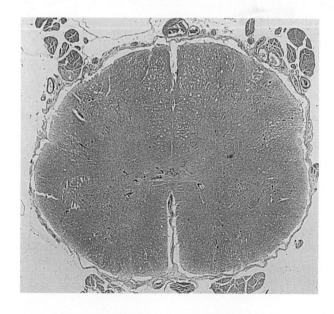

Figure 278   HIV myelopathy. Vacuolar myelopathy. (From Nelson JS, Parisi JE, Schochet SS Jr (Eds.). Principles and Practice of Neuropathology. St. Louis, MO: Mosby, 1993:95. With permission.)

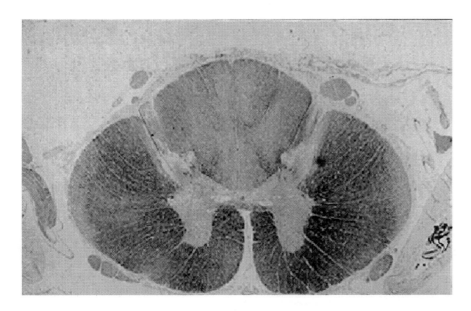

*Figure 279   Freidrich's ataxia (LFB).
Degeneration of axons and myelin in the
posterior columns and ventral spinocerebellar tracts (corticospinal tracts may also
be involved).*

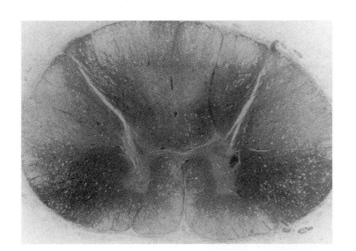

*Figure 280   Subacute combined degeneration (LFB). Spongy
degeneration of predominantly the posterior and lateral columns.*

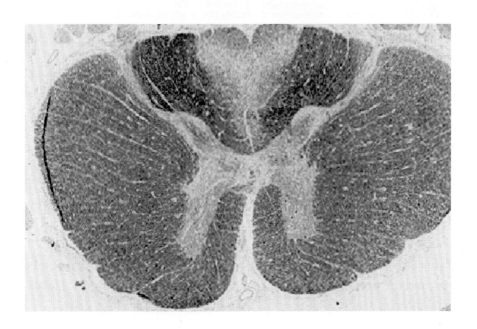

*Figure 281   Tabes dorsalis (LFB). Poste-
rior column demyelination.*

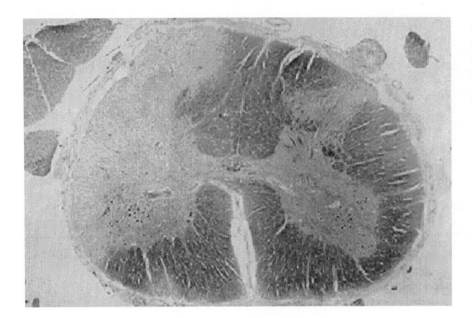

Figure 282   Multiple sclerosis (MS) (LFB). Demyelinative plaques extend across spinal cord tract boundaries involving lateral and dorsal columns and central gray.

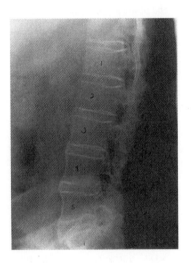

Figure 283   Ankylosing spondy-litis. Lateral x-ray demonstrates "Bamboo spine".

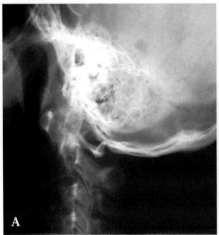

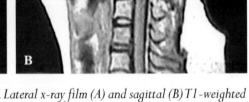

Figure 284   Rheumatoid arthritis pannus. Lateral x-ray film (A) and sagittal (B) T1-weighted MRI with a C1/2 pannus and anterior subluxation.

calcifications. X-ray films may demonstrate **"bamboo spine"** and zygapophyseal joint fusion. It is associated with uveitis and conjuctivitis (**Fig. 283**).

2. Rheumatoid arthritis—an autoimmune disease causing neurologic symptoms by necrotizing parenchymal vasculitis, leptomeningeal rheumatoid nodules, **pannus formation, atlanto–axial instability** (by transverse atlantoaxial ligament weakness), subaxial subluxations, and cranial settling. Eighty percent of cases affect the spine. It also affects the metatarso-phalangeal joints, metacarpo-phalangeal joints, and the proximal interphalangeal joints (Bouchard's nodes). Heberden's nodes form at the distal interphalangeal joints with degenerative arthritis (**Fig. 284**).

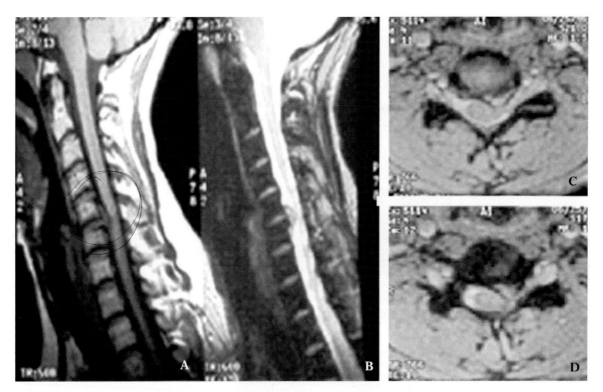

Figure 285   Herniated cervical disc. Sagittal T1 (A) and T2-weighted (B) and axial T2-weighted (C and D) MRIs demonstrate the left paracentral C5/6 herniation.

XXVIII. SPINAL DEGENERATIVE DISEASES

A. Eighty percent of adults will have an episode of lower back pain at some time in their lives.

B. Intervertebral disc disease

    1. In the lumbar spine 90% are at **L5/S1** and L4/5 and in the cervical spine 70% are at **C6/7** and 25% at C5/6.

    2. Most disc herniations are paracentral or central and 3% are foraminal and 4% are far-lateral. Rarely a herniated disc may be intradural. Thoracic discs account for <1% of herniated discs and 15% of these are asymptomatic (**Figs. 285 through 287**).

    3. With aging, discs lose water and proteoglycans and accumulate collagen. Annular tears may be concentric, radial (most frequent), or transverse.

    4. The discs are weakest posteriorly between the posterior longitudinal ligament (PLL) fibers. A lumbar disc bulge is seen in 35% of the normal population 20 to 39 years and in almost all patients >60 years. Asymptomatic herniations are seen in 33% of people >60 years.

    5. Herniated discs may have **peripheral enhancement**. Epidural postoperative fibrosis **enhances diffusely**. The DRG and posterior roots may enhance because there is no BBB.

    6. A **Schmorl's node** is a disc herniation through the end plate and is seen in 75% of the normal population.

    7. A vacuum disc forms by nitrogen accumulation with degenerative disease.

    8. The herniated disc was first described by Mixter and Barr in 1934.

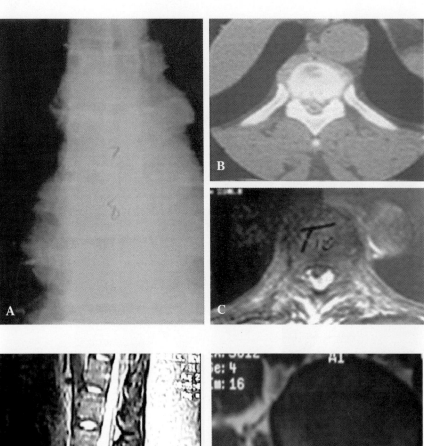

Figure 286   Herniated thoracic disc. AP thoracic x-ray film (A) and axial CT (B) demonstrate the calcified central T7/8 herniation. An axial T2-weighted MRI (C) demonstrates a soft T10/11 herniation.

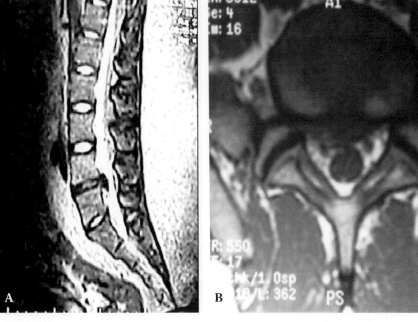

Figure 287   Herniated lumbar disc. Sagittal (A) T2-weighted and axial T1-weighted (B) MRIs demonstrate the L4/5 herniation.

C. Spondylosis

   1. It is most common after 50 years and affects 70% of the population > 50 years.

   2. When the discs degenerate, the bones rub against each other and elicit spurring. It is especially common at C5/6 (25%) and C6/7 (70%) because of increased mobility at these levels. Osteophytes develop near Sharpey's fibers where the anulus is connected to bone. Lumbar stenosis is usually due to hypertrophy of the superior articulating process (**Fig. 288**).

   3. The normal cervical spine diameter is 18 mm, and symptoms usually develop when it is < 10 mm.

   4. Symptoms are caused by microtrauma to the spinal cord (sliding up and down with flexion/extension and compression) and ischemia.

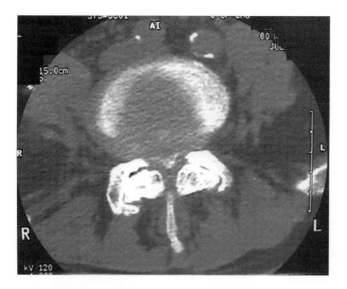

Figure 288   Lumbar stenosis. Axial CT demonstrates hypertrophic facets and thickened ligamentum flavum causing thecal sac compression.

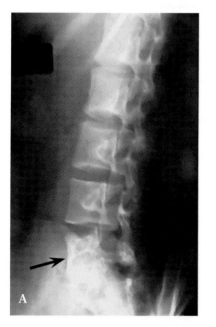
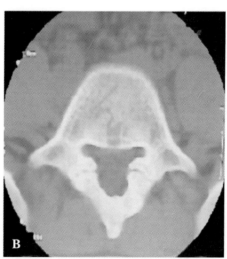
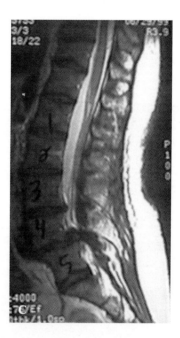

Figure 289   Spondylolisthesis. Oblique lumbar x-ray film (A) demonstrating the L5 "scotty dog with broken neck" (arrow) and (B) axial CT demonstrating the sclerotic pars defect of lytic spondylolisthesis. (C) Lateral T1-weighted MRI demonstrating L4/5 grade 1 spondylolisthesis.

5. The first case of cervical spondylosis was described by Brain in 1948.

D. Congenital spinal stenosis (short pedicle syndrome)—seen with achondroplasia and Morquioi's syndrome.

E. Spondylolysis—caused by a pars defect and seen in 5% of the population.

F. Spondylolisthesis—slippage of one vertebral body over another. It may be congenital, isthmic, pathologic, degenerative, or traumatic. Sixty-six percent occur at L4/5 and 30% at L5/S1 (**Figs. 289 through 291**).

G. Ossified posterior longitudinal ligament (OPLL)—more common in **Japan** and usually affects C3-5 and T4-7. Ossified ligamentum flavum also occurs in Japan (**Fig. 292**).

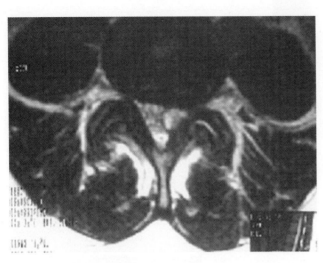

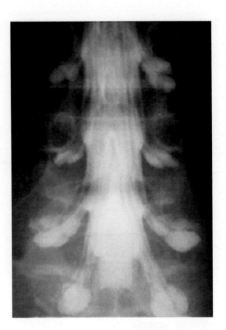

Figure 290   Synovial cyst. Axial T2-weighted MRI demonstrates a cyst emerging from the left facet joint.

Figure 291   Tarlov's cyst. AP myelogram demonstrates the multiple nerve sleeve dilations.

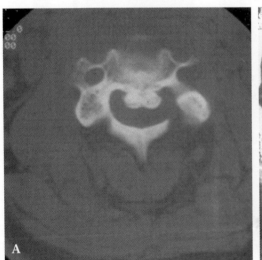

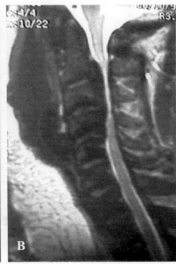

Figure 292   Ossified posterior longitudinal ligament. Axial CT bone window (A) and sagittal T2-weighted MRI (B) demonstrate C2-5 PLL calcification with cord compression.

H. Arachnoiditis—arachnoid collagen scar formation tethering nerve roots. It occurs after surgery, infection, intrathecal contrast, trauma, hemorrhage, and degenerative disease (**Fig. 293**).

I. Failed back surgery syndrome (FBSS)—possible causes include arachnoiditis, epidural fibrosis, hematoma, disc disease, infection, facet arthrosis, and referred hip pain. Most authorities believe that it is not helped by scar resection. FBSS is associated with enhancing roots after 6 months because the intradural roots should not enhance.

J. Syringomyelia

1. Ninety percent are associated with **Chiari I malformation** but they also occur with tumors, infections, and trauma.

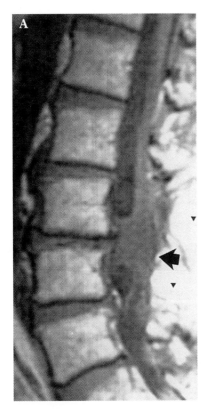

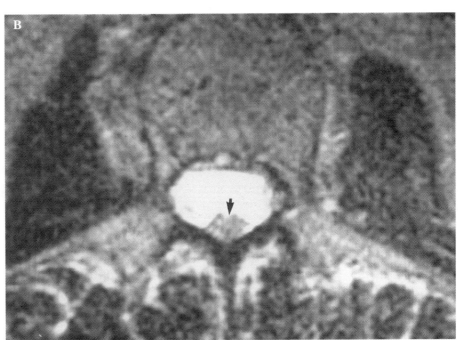

Figure 293   Arachnoiditis. Sagittal T1-weighted non-infused (A) and axial T2-weighted (B) MRIs demonstrating clumped and scarred nerve roots.

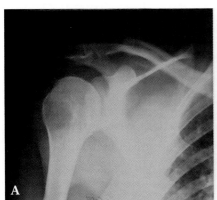
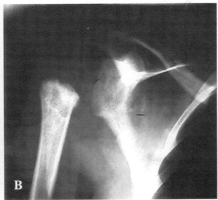

Figure 294   Charcot joint. AP shoulder x-ray film (A) is normal and (B) demonstrates complete erosion of the humeral head.

2. It is most commonly **cervical**. Onset is 35 to 45 years. It causes pain, **LMN findings in the UE and UMN finding in the LE** and a **capelike** loss of pain and temperature sensation (by damage to the spinothalamic fibers crossing in the anterior commissure).

3. It is also associated with **Charcot joints** (neuropathic osteoarthropathy) with a lytic humeral head or hypertrophic hip. These are usually seen with diabetes (in the foot or knee), syphilis (tabes dorsalis), MS, and leprosy. A Charcot shoulder joint is highly suspicious for a cervical syrinx (see Fig. 11 and **Fig. 294**).

4. Gardner hypothesized the "hydrodynamic theory" in which the choroid plexus systolic pumping forced CSF through the obex and patent central canal in the presence of an occluded foramen of Magendie and Luschka.

5. Williams hypothesized the "cranial-spinal dissociation theory" in which the pulse pressure transmitted through the epidural veins does not dissipate as quickly in the spine as it does in the brain and thus compresses the epidural space, cord, and syrinx producing "sloshing," with flow moving both rostrally and caudally.

6. Oldfield hypothesized that the CSF entered the syrinx cavity by way of the Virchow-Robin spaces and is pushed caudally with a pulse or Valsalva's maneuver, thus decreasing the syrinx width during Valsalva's maneuver or systole.

K. Morquio's syndrome (MPS4)—associated with a hypoplastic dens that may cause cord compression. Also, other MPSs are associated with thickened dura that may cause cord compression.

L. Achondroplasia—associated with increased periosteal bone and **short pedicles** (especially thoracolumbar) with frequent stenosis. It is also associated with hydrocephalus.

XXIX. SPINAL TRAUMA

A. Spinal shock—loss of spinal reflexes, sympathetic control and bladder function with ileus, flaccidity, and complete sensory loss that may last 1 to 6 weeks. The bulbocavernous reflex is usually the first to return. It may be due to loss of the descending influences that tonically excite lower neurons, rendering them closer to depolaration and more ready to respond. See Chapter II.

B. Hyperreflexia may develop after spinal shock resolves and includes Babinski responses, triple flexion responses, and spasticity of the bowel and bladder. The mass reflex is a complete autonomic discharge that includes urination, defecation, etc. Autonomic dysreflexia may develop where a stimulus such as a distended bladder may cause the levels of NE and EPI to increase causing hypertension, tachycardia, etc.

C. Anterior cord syndrome—due to severe flexion injury and causes hypesthesia (anterior spinothalamic tract), hypalgesia (lateral spinothalamic tract), and spastic paralysis (corticospinal tract). Posterior column function is retained.

D. Central cord syndrome—classically due to a hyperextension injury in a patient with a **narrow cervical spinal canal**. Symptoms and signs include decreased posterior column function, decreased sensation over the arms and shoulders, and weakness of the **UE** > **LE** (the UEs are more medial in the corticospinal tract).

E. **Brown-Sequard syndrome**—decreased contralateral pain and temperature, decreased ipsilateral proprioception, and ipsilateral hemiplegia. It is usually caused by a penetrating injury.

F. Primary injury—caused by concussion (transient decreased function), contusion, laceration, and compression.

G. Secondary injury—caused by ischemia, infection, hypoxia, hyperthermia, edema, hemorrhage, arachnoiditis, persistent compression, and syrinx. The syrinx is thought to form by progressive tearing from increased venous back pressure from Valsalva's maneuver on the spinal cord that is no longer mobile because of adhesions. Patients with nonpenetrating cervical cord injury should be treated with **methylprednisolone 30 mg/kg over 1 hour, followed by 5.4 mg/kg/h for 23 hours if started within 8 hours of the injury to help decrease secondary injury**. GM_1 ganglioside 100 mg IV qd has also been tested in a clinical trial.

H. Common traumatic spinal injuries—fracture-dislocation, fracture, and dislocation (3 : 1 : 1).

I. Most frequent levels involved—C1/2, C4-6, and T11-L2.

J. Thoracic injuries—less common because of high facets and ribs (decrease motion) and more canal space (no cervical and lumbar enlargements).

K. Flexion injuries—wedge fractures and dislocations.

L. Extension injuries—posterior element fractures.

M. Axial loading —compression, burst, and pillar fractures.

N. Rotational injuries—lateral mass fractures, unilateral facet subluxation, and uncovertebral fractures.

O. C1 injuries

1. Atlanto-occipital dislocation—frequently fatal. The dens-basion distance is > 12.5 mm (**Fig. 295**).

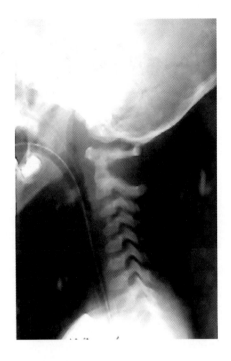

Figure 295   Atlanto-occipital and atlantoaxial dislocations. Lateral cervical spine x-ray film demonstrates increased distance from the occiput to the atlas and the atlas to the axis.

2. Jefferson fracture—bilateral burst fractures through the anterior and posterior neural arches. It is usually stable unless the transverse ligament is disrupted (**Fig. 296**).

3. Rotatory atlantoaxial subluxation—C1 is rotated over C2 > 45 degrees and the facets are locked. It is associated with flexion injuries, rheumatoid arthritis, and tonsillitis/pharyngitis (**Fig. 297**).

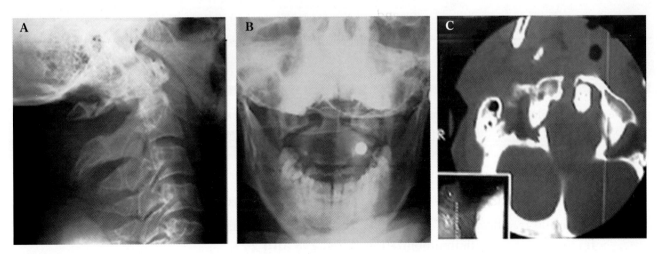

Figure 296   Jefferson fracture. Lateral (A) and open mouth (B) x-ray films and axial CT (C) demonstrate anterior and posterior arch fractures with prominent right-sided overhang seen in (B).

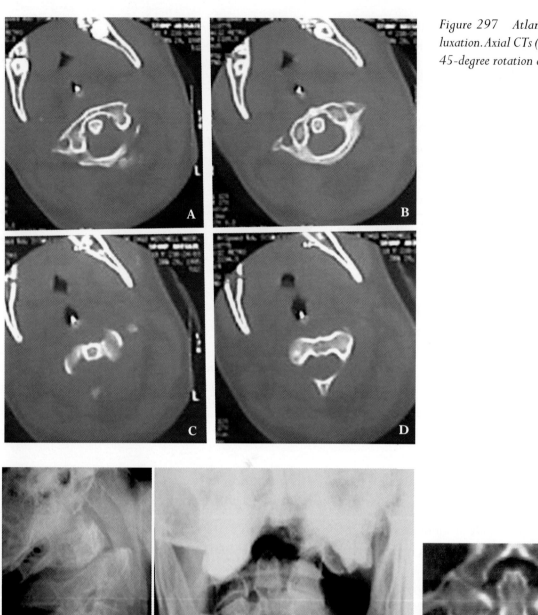

Figure 297   Atlanto-axial rotatory sub-luxation. Axial CTs (A to D) demonstrate the 45-degree rotation of the atlas on the axis.

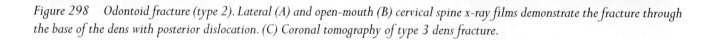

Figure 298   Odontoid fracture (type 2). Lateral (A) and open-mouth (B) cervical spine x-ray films demonstrate the fracture through the base of the dens with posterior dislocation. (C) Coronal tomography of type 3 dens fracture.

P.   C2 injuries

    1.   Odontoid fracture type 1—a fracture at the tip of the dens.

    2.   Odontoid fracture type 2—a fracture at the base of the dens. It is the least likely of the dens fractures to heal with immobilization (**Figs. 298 and 299**).

    3.   Odontoid fracture type 3—a fracture through the base of the axis body.

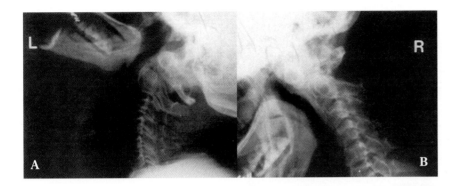

Figure 299   Os odontoideum. Lateral extension (A) and flexion (B) x-rays demonstrating an old dens defect with instability.

4. Hangman's fracture—C2 traumatic spondylolisthesis with bilateral pedicle fractures caused by hyperextension. It rarely causes cord injury (**Fig. 300**).

Q. C3-7 injuries

1. Flexion—wedge fracture (may disrupt interspinous and posterior longitudinal ligaments), facet fracture/dislocation, Clay shoveler's fracture (C6-T1 spinous process), and tear drop fracture (**Figs. 301 through 304**).

2. Extension—disrupts the anterior longitudinal ligament and causes an avulsion fracture of the anterior edge of the vertebral body and facet fracture.

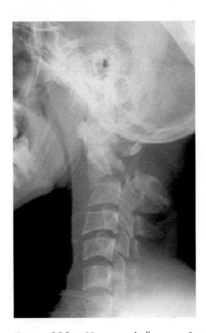

Figure 300   Hangman's fracture. Lateral cervical spine x-ray film demonstrates the C2 traumatic spondylolithesis with anterior angulation.

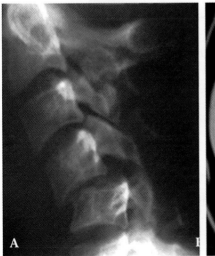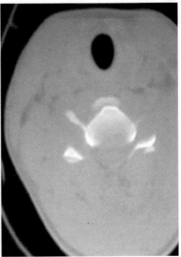

Figure 301   Unilateral interfacetal dislocation. Lateral cervical spine x-ray film (A) and axial CT (B) demonstrate the rotation with the left superior articulating process of C5 now dorsal to the inferior articulating process of C4.

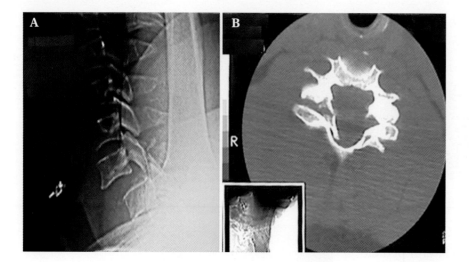

Figure 302   Bilateral interfacetal dislocation. Lateral cervical x-ray film (A) and axial CT (B) demonstrates the C6/7 injury with bilateral jumped facets.

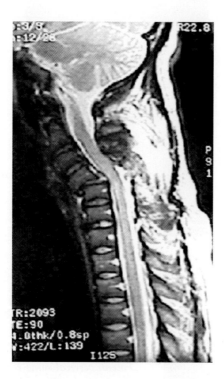

Figure 303   Flexion dislocation. Sagittal T2-weighted MRI demonstrates the C4/5 subluxation and angulation.

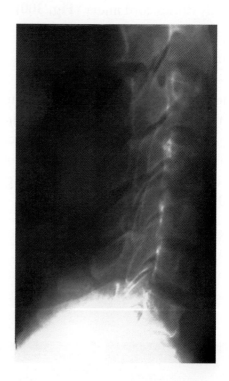

Figure 304   Clay shoveler's fracture. Lateral cervical x-ray film demonstrating C6 spinous process fracture.

R. Thoracic injuries—compression or burst fractures. They are usually stable (**Fig. 305**).

S. Thoracolumbar junction injuries—75% are compression injuries with anterior wedge fractures and intact posterior elements. Twenty percent are fracture dislocations.

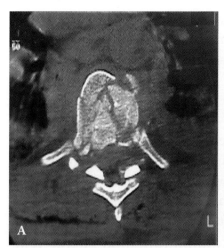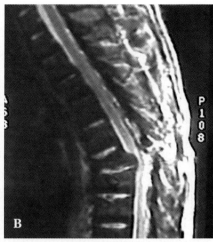

Figure 305   Burst fracture. Axial CT (A) and sagittal T2-weighted MRI (B) demonstrate angulation with retropulsion at T9.

XXX. PERIPHERAL NERVE DISORDERS

A. Etiologies—"DANG THE RAPIST." Diabetes and drugs, Alcohol, Neoplasm and nutritional, Guillian-Barré disease, Trauma, Hereditary, Electrolytes and endocrine, Renal, Amyloid and AIDS, Porphyria, Immune and ischemic, Sarcoid, and Toxins.

B. Sural nerve specimens are stained with H and E, trichrome (for connective tissue), and silver (for axons).

C. Peripheral nerves should contain three times more unmyelinated than myelinated fibers.

D. Amyloid affects the small fibers, whereas uremia affects the large fibers.

E. Wallerian degeneration—occurs **distal to the site of damage** after several days. The soma undergoes chromatolysis with increased protein synthesis. Retraction balls form from the build-up of transported material at the proximal and distal ends of cut nerves. All of the fascicles are at same stage of degeneration/regeneration and after regeneration the nodes are at regular intervals.

F. Bands of Bungner—proliferation of Schwann cells under the old basal lamina of a nerve with axons rowing inside.

G. **Segmental demyelination**—scattered demyelination with replacement by thinner myelin and shorter variable internodes (normally the nodes of Ranvier have a set internodal length). There is relative axonal sparing.

H. Secondary demyelination—only demyelination over certain axons (as with uremia) from axonal degeneration or wallerian degeneration distal to an injury (starts after 3 to 4 days).

I. Toxic neuropathy

  1. Axonal transport—affected by diabetes (decreases turnaround transport), vincristine/vinblastine (microtubles), mercury (translation), actinomycin D (transcription), and dinitrophenol (oxidative phosphorylation).

2. Schwann cells and myelin—affected by lead (bilateral wristdrop, see section XIII), diphtheria toxin (toxin inhibits Schwann cell myelin synthesis mainly in the DRG and ventral and dorsal roots where the blood-nerve barrier is normally absent, causes segmental demyelination without inflammation), and hexachlorophene.

J. Metabolic neuropathy

1. Diabetes mellitus—most frequently causes a **symmetric sensorimotor polyneuropathy** with stocking-glove decreased sensation and loss of myelin and axons. The neuropathy has multiple causes including increased glucose transport into axons, decreased intracellular transport, and hypoxia/ischemia. It may also cause a **focal mononeuropathy resulting from ischemia**. Diabetes also affects the autonomic nervous system.

2. Amyloid—extracellular β-pleated sheets form from **immunoglobulin light chains**. With Congo red staining, there is green birefringence with polarized light. It causes axonal degeneration with myelin destruction. Symptoms involve mainly autonomic dysfunction and loss of pain and temperature.

3. Porphyria—rapid, severe, symmetric, motor $>$ sensory loss, bilateral brachial weakness, and tachycardia, abdominal pain, psychiatric changes, and seizures. Autosomal dominant form is associated with acute intermittent porphyria and the attack may resolve in a few weeks. Death is by cardiac or respiratory causes. Axons and myelin are damaged and there is no inflammation. The liver defect causes a buildup of δ-aminolevulinic acid and porphobilinogen and the urine turns dark as it oxidizes. Treatment is with vitamin B_6, glucose, β-blockers, and hematin.

4. Others—uremia (painless, symmetric, sensorimotor, LE $>$ UE), leukodystrophy (MLD and Krabbe's disease affect both central and peripheral myelin), Fabry's disease, vitamin deficiencies, and hypothyroidism.

K. Autoimmune neuropathy

1. Cell-mediated immunity

    (a) Guillain-Barré (idiopathic polyneuritis) disease

    (i) It is one of the most frequent and most fatal neuropathies. It causes an acute inflammatory polyneuropathy with rapid onset. It affects all ages, has unknown cause, and is associated with trauma, surgery, infection, immunization, and neoplasm.

    (ii) It is usually monophasic peaking in 10 to 14 days but occasionally relapsing.

    (iii) It involves the DRG, ventral and dorsal nerve roots, and peripheral nerves causing mainly **motor and autonomic dysfunction** with less marked sensory symptoms. **Symmetric** weakness starts in the LE and moves cranially, progressing over 2 weeks.

    (iv) Pathologic examination demonstrates perivascular mononuclear infiltrates and **segmental demyelination**. The CSF reveals normal pressure, acellularity (90%), and increased protein after 5 weeks (initially normal).

    (v) NCV study demonstrates decreased velocity and amplitude.

    (vi) The mechanism may be due to cell-mediated immunity to myelin basic protein P2 in the peripheral myelin, due to humoral immunity, or due to a viral cause.

(vii) Differentiate from poliomyelitis (fever, asymmetric, no sensory findings), myasthenia gravis (no sensory finding and fatiguability), and botulism (abnormal pupillary reflexes and decreased heart rate).

(viii) Most recover with supportive care. Mortality is 3% and is usually due to cardiac arrest or respiratory problems. Ten percent have severe permanent weakness. Improvement may occur for up to 2 years. Three percent have a relapse.

(ix) Treatment is with plasmapheresis in the first 3 weeks to lessen the attack duration and severity if ambulation or respiration is in jeopardy. **It does not respond to steroids.**

(b) Experimental allergic neuritis—caused by T-cell–mediated attack of the P2 protein.

2. Humoral immunity—multiple causes.

L. Ischemic neuropathy (the vessel disease must be very severe because there are multiple anastomoses around nerves)

1. Polyarteritis nodosa (necrotizing panarteritis)—the most common necrotic vasculitis with CNS lesions. It affects small and medium-sized arteries throughout the body and causes polyneuropathy that may be symmetric or asymmetric (**mononeuropathy multiplex**) by obliteration of the vaso nervorum. It is associated with microaneurysms (70%), stenosis, and thrombosis. There is axonal degeneration and the vessel walls have intimal proliferation and inflammation with PMNs, lymphocytes, plasma cells, and eosinophils. Nodosa means segmental inflammation. It also causes skin purpura and renal dysfunction.

2. Collagen vascular disease.

3. Paraneoplastic syndrome—usually distal, sensorimotor, peaks in months and remains 1 to 2 years until death. The anti-Hu antibody is associated with oat cell pulmonary carcinoma and causes a sensory neuropathy involving the DRG.

M. Infectious neuropathy—the perineurium usually protects the nerve from the infectious process, but the overlying feeding vessel is at risk. Causes include varicella-zoster (may cause hemorrhagic ganglioradiculitis and rarely myelopathy), HIV, and leprosy (large swollen nerves in the distal extremities where it is cooler, ulnar nerve at the elbow and peroneal nerve at the fibular head).

N. Hereditary/hypertrophic (**onion bulb**) neuropathy

1. It occurs after demyelination/remyelination and has interspersed layers of Schwann cell processes and collagen. Nerves may be palpably enlarged. The NCV is decreased (**Figs. 306 through 308**).

2. Charcot-Marie-Tooth disease—autosomal **dominant** inheritance with onset in adolescence. It causes **peroneal muscle atrophy** and also degeneration of anterior horn cells, posterior columns, DRG, axons, and myelin. Distal muscle atrophy occurs in the feet and then the hands (develop claw hand). There is sensory ataxia and weakness **without autonomic dysfunction**. The CSF is normal.

3. Dejerine-Sottas disease—autosomal **recessive** inheritance and occurs < 10 years. It is slowly progressive with development of claw feet and hands, symmetric weakness, wasting of distal limbs, foot pain and paresthesias, without autonomic dysfunction. There is axon loss and **enlarged nontender ulnar, median, radial, and peroneal nerves**.

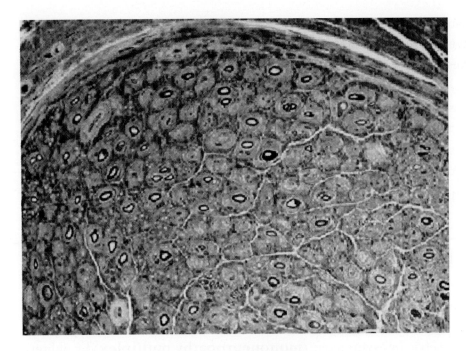

Figure 306   Onion-bulb formation (semithin epon section of osmicated sural nerve stained with toluene blue). Layers of Schwann cells and processes form around the axons.

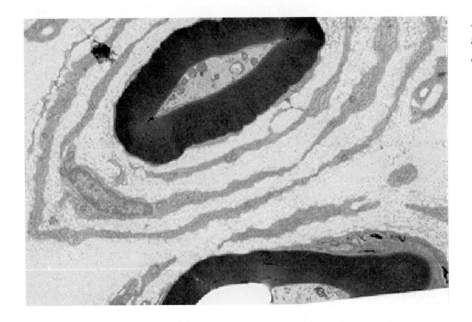

Figure 307   Onion-bulb formation (electron micrograph). Layers of Schwann cells and processes form around the axons.

4. Refsum's disease—autosomal **recessive** inheritance with onset in late childhood-early adulthood. There is a deficiency of phytanic acid oxidase with **accumulation of phytanic acid**. There is distal symmetric sensorimotor loss in LEs, and associated with retinitis pigmentosum, cardiomyopathy, and hearing loss.

5. Chronic inflammatory demyelinating polyradiculopathy—may be a chronic form of Guillain-Barré syndrome.

6. Others—lead, Krabbe's disease, and metachromatic leukodystrophy.

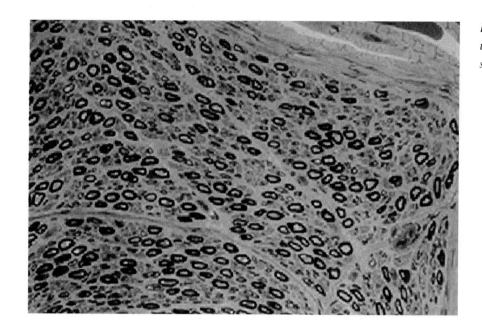

Figure 308 Normal sural nerve (semi-thin epon section of osmicated sural nerve stained with toluene blue).

O. Traumatic neuropathy

    1. Neuropraxia—there is functional but no structural damage (nerve concussion) with temporary loss of function that may last 6 to 8 weeks. Motor function is affected more than sensation.

    2. Axonotmesis—interuption of axons and myelin with intact perineurium and epineurium. Spontaneous regeneration may occur at 1 to 2 mm/d.

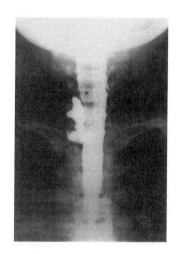

    3. Neurotmesis—complete transection of the nerve and nerve sheath. Axonal regeration may lead to neuroma formation (**Fig. 309**).

Figure 309 Brachial plexus avulsion.

P. Motor deficits—By nutritional, metabolic, Guillain-Barré syndrome and toxic causes. It is usually symmetric in the distal LEs (affects the longest and largest nerves).

Q. Sensory deficits—by amyloid and toxic causes. It is usually symmetric distal limb LE > UE and affects all modalities, but vibration is usually the most sensitive.

R. Paresthesias/dysesthesias—due to diabetes and ETOH. They are from ectopic impulse transmission in damaged nerves.

S. Autonomic deficits—secondary to amyloid, diabetes, Shy-Drager syndrome and small fiber polyneuropathies.

T.   Toxins—tend to cause sensory > motor deficits, whereas Guillain-Barré tends to cause motor > sensory deficits.

U.   Evaluation of neuropathy

  1. Mononeuropathy versus polyneuropathy versus mononeuropathy multiplex versus plexus injury.

  2. Motor > sensory (Guillain-Barré syndrome diphtheria, porphyria, uremia), sensory > motor (ETOH, arsenic, lead, and INH), or pure motor, sensory, or autonomic.

  3. Time course—rapid (vascular, toxic, inflammation, immune), subacute (toxic, nutritional, systemic), and slow (hereditary, metabolic).

  4. Axonal versus myelin degeneration.

  5. Diagnostic tests include EMG/NCV, CSF studies, nerve and muscle biopsies, and biochemical studies.

V.   Mononeuritis multiplex (subacute asymmetric polyneuropathy)

  1. Diabetes—acute ophthalmoplegia (**CN III nerve palsy, sudden onset, spares pupil, lesion in center of nerve, usually painful, and often recovers well**), acute ischemic femoral neuropathy (recovers well), progressive distal symmetric sensory loss (most common), symmetric or asymmetric motor with or without sensory loss, autonomic loss, and pain dysesthesia syndromes. The mechanism is ischemia of the vaso nervorum with segmental demyelination.

  2. Ischemia and vasculitis.

W.   Morton's neuroma—a traumatic neuroma that forms on the digital nerve between the toes.

X.   Neonates—may have a plexus injury involving C5 and 6 (**Erb's palsy**, arms hang at side with a normal hand) or C7, C8, and T1 (**Klumpke's palsy**, clawhand with wasting, occasional Horner's syndrome).

Y.   Brachial plexitis—idiopathic onset of upper limb pain and weakness that usually resolves in 6 to 12 weeks. There is no fever, leukocytosis, or increased ESR. The cause is unclear (CMV, AIDS, unknown). Mononuclear cells may be seen in the nerve fascicles.

Z.   Carpal tunnel syndrome—distal median neuropathy caused by compression at the wrist from the transverse carpal ligament. There is female predominance. 50% are bilateral. It usually is more severe in the dominant hand and causes wasting of the thenar eminence, weakness of the flexor pollicis brevis, adductor pollicis, opponens pollicis, abductor pollicis brevis, sensory loss of the thumb and first finger, and nocturnal paresthesias. It is associated with **multiple myeloma, amyloid, rheumatoid arthritis, acromegaly, mucopolysaccharidoses, hypothyroidism, and pregnancy**. A pronator syndrome is caused by median nerve compression between the heads of the pronator teres.

AA. Ulnar neuropathy—may cause **clawhand** with extension at the metacarpophalangeal joint and flexion at the interphalangeal joint of the fourth and fifth digits because of decreased function of the lumbricals. Lumbricals 2 and 3 are innervated by the median nerve. Cubital tunnel syndrome is caused by compression of the ulnar nerve under the two heads of the flexor carpi ulnaris.

BB. Posterior interosseous syndrome—weakness of the radially innervated forearm and hand muscles (supinator, extensor digitorum, extensor carpi ulnaris, and abductor pollicis) and **decreased sensation** of the dorsolateral forearm and hand. It causes a fingerdrop without a wristdrop because of sparing of the extensor carpi ulnaris.

CC. Anterior interosseus syndrome—pure weakness **without sensory loss** caused by compression of the anterior interosseus branch of the median nerve in the deep forearm. It involves the pronator quadratus, flexor pollicis longus and flexor digitorum profundus 2 and 3 (FDP 4 and 5 are innervated by the ulnar nerve).

DD. Meralgia paresthetica—compression of the **lateral femoral cutaneous nerve** (L2,3) under the inguinal ligament. It causes anterolateral thigh numbness and dysesthesia. It is associated with obesity, pregnancy, and diabetes.

EE. Tarsal tunnel syndrome—compression of the tibial nerve with paresthesias of the sole of the foot without motor changes.

FF. Reflex sympathetic dystrophy (RSD)—an abnormal response of the **sympathetic** nervous system that develops after trauma or an incomplete peripheral nerve injury. It is associated with sudomotor, vasomotor, and trophic changes: **causalgia** (a persistent burning pain that is elicited by contact, pain, temperature changes, and emotion), limb cyanosis and coldness, and **Sudek's atrophy** (atrophy of the bone, joints, muscle, and skin **without nerve atrophy**). The skin is smooth and shiny. RSD develops after a partial tear of a nerve and may be due to an abnormal connection of efferent and afferent sympathetic fibers. Treatment is with anti-sympathetic medications or sympathectomy.

GG. Facial nerve diseases

1. Bell's palsy—causes unilateral CN VII dysfunction with sudden onset. The cause is unknown though it is possibly viral. Weakness peaks in 2 to 5 days. There may also be decreased taste and sensation and hyperacusis. 80% recover completely. Treatment is with steroids for 1 week, and prevention of corneal damage due to inability to close the eye and decreased lacrimation.

2. Ramsay Hunt syndrome—herpes zoster infection of the geniculate ganglion with CN VII dysfunction, possibly CN VIII dysfunction, and vesicular lesions of the ear.

3. Bilateral CN VII nerve palsy—Guillain-Barré disease and Lyme disease.

4. Supranuclear lesions—spare the upper face because of its bilateral innervation and may be associated with dissociation of emotional and voluntary lower face movements.

5. Hemifacial spasm—intermittent spasms of the CN VII muscles. Onset 40 to 60 years with **female** predominance. **Spasms start near the eye** and move caudally. It is possibly caused by segmental demyelination with ephatic transmission. Treatment is with microvascular decompression (the AICA is usually the artery that compresses CN VII), carbamozepine (Tegretol), or Botox injections q5 months.

6. Adies syndrome—degeneration of the **ciliary ganglion** and postganglionic parasympathetic fibers. There is female predominance. It causes paralysis of the pupillary sphincter with mydriasis. The **pupil responds better to near than light** (also with syphilis and Parinaud's syndrome), and the pupil constricts with 0.1% pilocarpine.

XXXI. NEUROMUSCULAR JUNCTION DISEASES

A. Myasthenia gravis (MG)

    1. It affects two populations: **30-year-old women** (most common) and **60-year-old men with thymomas**. Ten percent of cases have a thymoma but 80% have thymic hyperplasia.

    2. Symptoms begin with **extraocular weakness** and are worse with exertion and better with rest. Proximal muscles are affected more than distal and it is remitting/relapsing. Symptoms include ptosis, expressionless facies, and dysphagia. There is rarely muscle atrophy. The **pupillary response is retained**. The symptoms are caused by **antibodies to nicotinic ACh receptors** on the postsynaptic end plate, but **10 to 15% of cases do not have ACh-r Ig**.

    3. There is a **decremental EMG** (strength deteriorates with use) and a positive Tensilon test (using edrophonium).

    4. MG is associated with hyperthyroidism, RA, SLE, and polymyositis. Botulism may have a similar initial presentation but causes unreactive pupils. **Aminoglycosides** may worsen symptoms by decreasing the Ca^{++} flux at the NMJ.

    5. Treatment is with anticholinesterase medications (neostigmine or pyridostigmine), steroids, thymectomy, plasmapheresis, and azathioprine (immunosuppressant). Initial treatment is with anticholinesterase medications. If the dose is too high, a **"cholinergic crisis"** may develop with muscle weakness, salivation, diarrhea, bradycardia, miosis, sweating, and nausea/vomiting. Assess by giving endophronium: if the symptoms are worse or not improved, decrease the anticholinesterase dose. If the strength improves, increase the dose.

    6. Consider thymectomy if a thymoma is seen on CT, although $\frac{1}{3}$ of patients improve after thymectomy even when no thymoma is detected. If there are only ocular symptoms for $>$ 1 year, there is no need for thymectomy because most patients do very well. Thymectomy should be performed between puberty and 60 years.

    7. Steroids should be started after both anticholinesterases and thymectomy fail. Azathioprine may be used if prednisone is not tolerated. The final option is plasma exchange.

B. Eaton-Lambert syndrome (myasthenic syndrome)—an autoimmune Ig attack on the **presynaptic terminal** that decreases the area of the active zone and **decreases the number of ACh quanta released** by reducing the Ca^{++} ion entry into the presynaptic terminal. There is a **male predominance**. It causes **proximal limb fatigue**, has an **incremental EMG** (with strength improving at first with contractions), spares ocular and bulbar muscles, reduces reflexes, and **impairs autonomic function**. Sixty percent of cases are associated with pulmonary **oat cell carcinoma**. There is no response to anticholinesterase medications and there are no fasciculations. Treatment is with plasmapheresis, steroids, and immunosuppression. Symptoms may be improved with guanidine. The syndrome can be transferred to another patient with immunoglobulins.

C. Botox, aminoglycosides, increased Mg^{++}, and decreased Ca^{++} decrease the presynaptic ACh release.

XXXII. MUSCLE DISEASES

A. A muscle fiber contains multiple parallel myofibrils made up of sarcomeres (Z line to Z line). The nuclei are on the periphery of the cell, although they may be internal at the tendon junction or with myotonic dystrophy or centronuclear myopathy (see Chapter II).

1. **Type 1 muscle fibers** (red muscle)—increased mitochondria, aerobic metabolism, slower but more sustained action with less fatiguing, and used for posture.

2. **Type 2 muscle fibers** (white muscle)—less mitochondria, relies on anaerobic metabolism with glycolysis, quick action but fatiguable, more numerous then red muscle, and used for flight, and so forth.

3. **A band**—contains thick filaments with myosin and thin filaments with actin.

4. **I band**—contains thin filaments with actin.

5. **H band**—contains only thick filaments with myosin.

6. Muscle biopsy—demonstrates the number and size of fibers, storage diseases, segmental necrosis with regeneration (myositis), mosaic pattern changes (denervation), and the NMJ.

7. Type 1 fiber atrophy—myotonic dystrophy, congenital myopathy.

8. Type 2 fiber atrophy—myasthenia gravis, denervation, disuse, paraneoplastic syndrome, and steroids.

9. Type 1 hypertrophy—werdnig-Hoffman disease.

10. Type 2 hypertrophy—congenital fiber-type disproportion.

11. Nonselective atrophy—denervation (85% decrease in volume in 3 months).

12. Nonselective hypertrophy—limb-girdle dystrophy, myotonia congenita, acromegaly.

B. Congenital myopathies usually—cause a mild disability, are nonprogressive, and are more severe proximally. Includes central core disease, multicore disease, nemaline rod myopathy, and myotubular myopathy.

C. Muscular dystrophy (MD)

1. Hereditary diseases causing degeneration of muscle with symmetric weakness with normal neural function. They usually cause progressive **proximal** weakness. The most common varieties are myotonic dystrophy and Duchenne's dystrophy. Evaluation should include serum CK, aldolase, and myoglobin, urine myoglobin, EMG, and muscle biopsy. In adults, the differential diagnosis includes polymyositis (more rapid course, higher CK than MD except Duchenne's dystrophy, which is only in children, more fibrillation potentials on EMG, and improvement with steroids) and spinal-muscular atrophy (usually younger, and with abnormal NCV). There is no treatment for MD, except for Duchenne's dystrophy for which prednisone may help. Quinine may help decrease the hypertonicity in myotonic MD. Old contractures can be treated with fasciotomy and tendon lengthening.

2. Congenital MD—autosomal recessive, weakness present at birth, more common in Japan, with or without mental retardation.

3. Duchenne's MD—the most common type. It is **X-linked recessive** but 30% are from spontaneous mutation. There is male predominance. It occurs in 1 in 3500 births and peak age is 2 to 5 years. There is rapid progression. There is **decreased dystrophin** that is needed to stabilize membranes. It causes **atrophy of the shoulder and pelvic girdles** and **pseudohypertrophy of the calf** with fatty and fibrous replacement. It starts in the lower trunk and then spreads to the lower extremity and later the proximal upper extremity with sparing of the hands, face, and eyes. Patients use Gower's maneuver to stand, have a waddling gait (from bilateral gluteus medius weakness), occasionally have **decreased IQ**, and are prone to **CHF and respiratory infections**. The serum **CK levels are very elevated** and peak at 3 years. Biopsy demonstrates muscle fiber necrosis and regeneration. Mortality is 75% by 25 years.

4. Becker's MD—X-linked recessive inheritance with male predominance that occurs in 1 in 30,000 births. It has a later onset (11 years), is a less severe version of Duchenne's MD, and there is **rarely CHF or mental retardation**. There is **abnormal dystrophin** and pseudohypertrophy, but no fiber necrosis and regeneration. Patients are nonambulatory by 30 years and usually die by 50 years.

5. Facioscapulohumeral dystrophy—**autosomal dominant** inheritance. The defect is located on **chromosome 4**. It is mild and slowly progressive with peak age 10 to 20 years. It involves the face, shoulder, and upper arm, and starts at the face and descends. There is no pseudohypertrophy, mental retardation, or CHF. There is sensorineural hearing loss. It is the **only MD with chronic inflammatory cells within the muscle**. There is no fiber necrosis or regeneration and the **serum CK is normal**. There is frequently **absence of a muscle**.

6. Limb-girdle syndrome—autosomal recessive inheritance with onset in childhood or early adulthood. There is slow progression with proximal axial weakness, frequent CHF but no mental retardation, and pseudohypertrophy in 33%.

7. Distal myopathy—multiple types.

8. Oculopharyngeal MD—autosomal dominant inheritance with peak age 45 years. The serum CK is normal. There is ptosis and dysphagia.

9. Myotonic MD—the **most common MD in adults** with **autosomal dominant** inheritance. The gene is located on **chromosome 19**. It occurs in 5 in 100,000 births and peak age is 30 years. It initially affects the **face and then the distal extremities** with weakness or myotonus first. The muscles are unable to relax after contraction. There are dysrhythmias, **decreased intelligence**, **cataracts** (90%), endocrine dysfunction (with testicular atrophy), and **frontal balding** in both sexes. They are usually nonambulatory within 20 years of disease onset. The congenital form is only inherited from the mother. The myotonia can be treated with quinine or procainamide (these may increase an AV block) or phenytoin (Dilantin).

D. Metabolic myopathies

1. They usually involve the proximal LE, rarely involve the face and eyes, and the serum CK is usually elevated.

2. Glycogen storage (in vacuoles).

(a) Acid maltase deficiency—autosomal recessive inheritance with glycogen storage in vacuoles. The infantile form is **Pompe's disease** with onset at 1 month and death by 2 years, hepatomegaly, and a cardiorespiratory death. Glycogen accumulates in the liver, heart, skeletal muscle, and motor neurons.

(b) McArdle's disease—autosomal recessive inheritance with **myophosphorylase deficiency**. Peak age at onset is 15 years. It is only symptomatic with increased activity, and causes myalgia, increased CK, and myoglobinuria.

(c) Phosphofructokinase deficiency—autosomal recessive inheritance with male predominance, and similar features to McArdle's disease.

(d) **Lafora's disease**—autosomal recessive inheritance with peak age 6 to 18 years. It is systemic, fatal, and causes seizures, decreased mentation, focal deficits, and affects the heart, liver, skin, nerves, and muscles with accumulation of Lafora's bodies (basophilic with dark center caused by the **intracellular accumulation** of polyglucosans).

3. Lipid storage (in vacuoles)

(a) Carnitine deficiency—inability to use long-chain fatty acids for metabolism. It may be systemic or muscular, and causes mild weakness.

(b) Fabry's disease—X-linked inheritance with deficiency of α-galactosidase and accumulation of ceramides. It causes peripheral nerve pain, decreased sweating, corneal opacities, renal insufficiency, and skin angiokeratomas.

4. Mitochondrial myopathy—ragged red muscle fibers caused by large subsarcolemal mitochondria. It is associated with retinal, ocular, and cardiac abnormalities. It is inherited from **maternal mitochondrial DNA**. Variants are MELAS, MERRF, Kearns-Sayre syndrome, and Luft's disease.

5. Malignant hyperthermia—autosomal dominant inheritance and occurs in 1 in 15,000 anesthetic procedures. The risk is increased with inhalation anesthetics (**halothane**) and **succinylcholine** in combination. The body temperature increases $1°$ C every five minutes and may reach $110°$ F. It is caused by increased muscle metabolism from sustained rigidity. There is increased O_2 use and lactate formation causing acidosis. Symptoms include tachycardia, dysrhythmia, hypertension or hypotension, hyperventilation, muscle rigidity, fever (50%), hyperkalemia, increased serum CK, myoglobinuria, and renal failure. There is a 70% mortality without treatment with **dantrolene**, 2.5 mg/kg IV q15min then 2 mg/kg PO QID for 3 days. Dantrolene acts by reducing the Ca^{++} release from the SR and reduces the mortality to 7%. Treatment also requires discontinuation of the anesthesia, cooling procedures, hydration, and intravenous sodium bicarbonate. The disease is related to a defect in a Ca^{++} release channel (ryanoidine receptor) with increased Ca^{++} release from the SR. Patients at highest risk have a family history, increased serum CK, and central core disease. Diagnose high-risk patients by the contracture test, see muscle contraction in vitro with exposure to caffeine or halothane.

6. Thyroid myopathy—chronic thyrotoxic myopathy (affects middle-aged males, weakness and wasting of proximal muscles), exophthalmic ophthalmoplegia (associated with Grave's disease, spares pupillary and ciliary function, painful, muscle is infiltrated with monocytes and lipocytes, **inferior and medial rectus are most affected**, impaired upgaze, and treatment is with

steroids), thyrotoxic periodic paralysis (treat with β-blockers), and hypothyroidism (stiff, slow, and swollen muscles) (**Fig. 310**).

7. Others—steroids, Addison's disease, and Cushing's disease.

E. Inflammatory myopathy

1. Bacterial myositis—usually caused by *Staphylococcus aureus*. The risk is increased with closed injuries. It causes fever, leukocytosis, and tenderness.

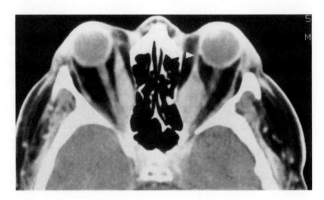

Figure 310   Thyroid ophthalmology. Axial CT demonstrating enlarged medial rectus muscles.

2. Trichinosis myositis—involves the eye, face, and proximal limbs. It causes a puffy face, muscle tenderness, and eosinophilia. Both muscle fiber types are involved. Treatment is with thiabendazole and prednisone. Parasitic myositis is also caused by toxoplasmosis and cysticercosis.

3. Viral myositis—usually caused by influenza and coxsackieviruses. It is seen in childhood epidemics. It is occasionally associated with rhabdomyolysis, ATN and renal failure. It resolves in 1 to 2 weeks. Viral myositis is also caused by HIV and HTLV.

4. Polymyositis—the most frequent inflammatory myopathy in adults with peak age 30 to 50 years and **female predominance**. It causes subacute, **painless**, symmetric, proximal more than distal, limb and trunk weakness with dysphagia, rare fever, malaise, and myalgia. It has a relapsing course with increased serum ESR and CK and urine myoglobinuria. More than 50% of cases are ANA positive and EMG positive. There are **T cells in the muscle fibers** with macrophages. Treatment is with steroids and physical therapy to prevent contractures. Ten percent are **associated with cancer**. The active phase of the disease lasts around 2 years, most people improve, 20% recover, and there is a 15% mortality.

5. Dermatomyositis—There is a **female predominance** and it occurs in children and adults. The initial symptom is a maculopapular skin rash: **butterfly lesion** over the face or on the eyelid with **periorbital edema (heliotrope** or lilac colored), or skin lesions on the neck, shoulders, and **extensors** of the extremities. The weakness is proximal and there is an angiopathy affecting skin, muscle, peripheral nerve, and intestines (causing ulcerations). The inflammation is **humoral with increased antibodies and C3**. There are **B lymphocytes around the vessels but not in the muscle fibers** as in polymyositis. Treatment is with steroids and physical therapy. Ten percent are **associated with cancer** and 30% also have Raynaud's syndrome. The active phase of the disease lasts around 2 years, most people improve, 20% recover, and there is a 15% mortality.

6. Inclusion body myositis—peak age is 60 years with a male predominance. It is slowly progressive, painless LE weakness, steroid resistant, normal CPK, and microscopy is similar to polymyositis but with intranuclear inclusions. It may be caused by a virus or prion.

7. Drug-induced inflammatory myopathies—caused by penicillamine and tryptophan. The CK is normal and there is perivascular eosinophils.

F. Miscellaneous

1. Rhabdomyolysis—destruction of striated muscle usually from ischemia or trauma. Myoglobin (smaller than hemoglobin and not bound to haptoglobin) enters the kidneys and may cause renal failure. There is fever, leukocytosis, pain, and albumin loss in the urine.

2. Familial periodic paralysis—due to a genetic defect coding for Na^+, Cl^-, or Ca^{++} channels in the muscle fiber membranes (most commonly related to Ca^{++} channels). There is autosomal dominant inheritance with a male predominance. It is characterized by intermittent episodes of paralysis with onset in late childhood and episodes occurring every few weeks, although the frequency decreases with age. Attacks are associated with hyperkalemia and hypokalemia, hyperthyroidism, and cold weather. It is diagnosed by a very low serum K^+ (1.8 mEq/dL) and weakness exacerbated by glucose, NaCl, and exercise that is relieved with KCl. The muscle sarcoplasm develops vacuoles. Treat with KCl, 5 to 10 g PO qd, imipramine, acetazolamide, and limiting carbohydrates and NaCl.

3. Muscle cramps—caused by sustained contraction after muscle stretching. It is associated with pregnancy, dehydration, hypothyroidism, and dialysis. It is improved by massage and stretching, and can be treated with quinine or diphenhydramine (Benadryl).

4. Energy is obtained from glycogen during exercise and from fatty acids/triglycerides during rest.

5. $K^+ < 2.5$ or > 9 mEq/dL—flaccid paralysis and decreased DTRs.

6. $Ca^{++} < 7$ mEq/dL (or with decreased P_{CO_2})—the muscles may overfire and cause tetany.

7. $Ca^{++} > 12$ mEq/dL—muscle weakness.

8. Hypermagnesemia—tetany.

9. Hypomagnesemia—weakness.

10. Serum CKmb (heart muscle), CKmm (skeletal muscle), and CKbb (nervous tissue). The "m" is for muscle and the "b" is for brain. CKmb $> 6\%$ suggests MI.

11. Muscle fibers increase or decrease in size with exercise, etc., but the number of cells does not change. Denervation occurs with aging and causes group atrophy.

12. Differential diagnosis of peripheral weakness syndromes

    (a) Ocular palsy (Spare pupil)—hyperthyroidism and myasthenia gravis.

    (b) Bilateral facial palsy—myasthenia gravis, fasciohumeroscapular muscular dystrophy, Guillain-Barré syndrome, and Lyme disease.

    (c) Bulbar palsy—myasthenia gravis and botulism.

    (d) Cervical weakness (inability to lift head)—idiopathic polymyositis.

    (e) Weakness of respiratory muscles and trunk—polymyositis, glycogen storage diseases, and motor system diseases.

    (f) Bilateral UE weakness—ALS.

    (g) Bilateral LE weakness—polyneuropathy.

    (h) Limb-girdle weakness—polymyositis, dermatomyositis, and MD. Duchenne MD (LE) and Landouzy-Dejerine dystrophy (face and shoulder).

    (i) Generalized weakness—familial hypokalemia/hyperkalemia.

    (j) Weakness of one muscle—neuropathy, seldom myopathy (except familial periodic paralysis).

Glossary

A

ACA	anterior cerebral artery
ACh	acetylcholine
ACOM	anterior communicating artery
ACTH	adrenocorticotropic hormone
ADH	antidiuretic hormone
AFB	acid-fast bacillus
AFP	alpha-fetoprotein
AICA	anterior inferior cerebellar artery
AIDS	acquired immune deficiency syndrome
ALD	adrenoleukodystrophy
ALL	acute lymphocytic leukemia
ALS	amyotrophic lateral sclerosis
ANA	antinuclear antibody
APUD	amine precursor uptake and decarboxylation
ARAS	ascending reticular activating system
ARDS	acute respiratory distress syndrome
ASA	acetylsalicylic acid (aspirin)
ATIII	antithrombin III
ATP	adenosine triphosphate
ATPase	adenosine triphosphatase
AVM	arteriovenous malformation
AZT	azidothymidine

B

BAER	brain stem auditory evoked response
BAL	2,3-dimercaptopropanol
BBB	blood-brain barrier
BCNU	carmustine
BMR	basal metabolic rate
BT	bleeding time
BUN	blood urea nitrogen

C

CAI	complete androgen insensitivity
CAM	cell adhesion molecule
CAMP	cyclic adenosine monophosphate
CBC	complete blood count
CBF	cerebral blood flow
CCA	common carotid artery
CCF	cavernous-carotid fistula
CCK	cholecystokinin
CEA	carcinoembryonic antigen
CHF	congestive heart failure
CJD	Creutzfeldt-Jakob disease
$CMRO_2$	cerebral metabolic rate of oxygen
CMV	cytomegalovirus
CN	cranial nerve
CNS	central nervous system
CPA	cerebellopontine angle
CPM	central pontine myelinosis
CPR	cardiopulmonary resuscitation
CRH	corticotropin-releasing hormone
CSF	cerebrospinal fluid
CT	computed tomography
CVA	cerebrovascular accident
CXR	chest x-ray

D

DA	dopamine
DAG	diacylglycerol
DAI	diffuse axonal injury
DDAVP	desmopressin acetate
DI	diabetes insipidus
DIC	disseminated intravascular coagulation

DKA	diabetic ketoacidosis
DNA	deoxyribonucleic acid
DOPA	dihydroxyphenylalanine (methyldopa)
DPG	2,3-diphosphoglycerate
DRG	dorsal root ganglion
DSC	dorsal spinocerebellar
DTR	deep tendon reflex
DVT	deep venous thrombosis

E

EAM	experimental allergic encephalomyelitis
EBV	Epstein-Barr virus
ECA	external carotid artery
ECG	electrocardiogram
EC-IC	external carotid-internal carotid
EDH	epidural hematoma
EDTA	ethylenediaminetetraacetic acid
EEG	electroencephalogram
EHL	extensor hallucis longus
ELISA	enzyme-linked immunosorbent assay
EMA	epithelial membrane antigen
EMG	electromyelogram
EPI	epinephrine
ER	endoplasmic reticulum
ESR	erythrocyte sedimentation rate
ETOH	ethanol

F

FBSS	failed back surgery syndrome
FFP	fresh frozen plasma
FMD	fibromuscular dysplasia
FSH	follicle-stimulating hormone

G

GABA	gamma-aminobutyric acid
GBM	glioblastoma multiforme
GCS	Glasgow coma scale

GDP	guanosine diphosphate
GFAP	glial fibrillary acidic protein
GH	growth hormone
GHIH	growth hormone-inhibiting hormone
GHRH	growth hormone-releasing hormone
GI	gastrointestinal
GM	granulocyte-macrophage
GNB	gram-negative bacilli
GnRH	gonadotropin-releasing hormone
GP	globus pallidus
GPe	globus pallidus externa
GPm	medial globus pallidus
GPi	globus pallidus interna
GTP	guanosine triphosphate
GU	genitourinary

H

Hb	hemoglobin
HCG	human chorionic gonadotropin
HDL	high-density lipoprotein
H & E	hematoxylin and eosin
HELLP	hemolysis, elevated liver enzymes, and low platelet count
HGPRT	hypoxanthine-guanine phosphoribosyltransferase
HIV	human immunodeficiency virus
HLA-DR2	human leukocyte antigen-DR2
HPF	high-power field
HSV	herpes simplex virus
5-HT	5-hydroxytryptamine (serotonin)
HTLV	human T-cell lymphotropic virus
HZV	herpes zoster virus

I

IC	internal capsule
ICA	internal carotid artery
ICH	intracranial hemorrhage

ICP	intracranial pressure	MERRF	myoclonus, epilepsy, and red-ragged fibers
IFN	interferon	MG	myasthenia gravis
Ig	immunoglobulin	MGB	medial geniculate body
INH	isoniazid	MI	myocardial infarction
INO	internuclear ophthalmoplegia	MID	multi-infarct dementia
IP$_3$	inositol 1,4,5-triphosphate	ML	medial lemniscus
IPH	intraparenchymal hemorrhage	MLD	metachromatic leukodystrophy
IQ	intelligence quotient	MLF	medial longitudinal fasciculus
ITP	idiopathic thrombocytopenic purpura	MM	multiple myeloma
IV	intravenous	MOF	multiple organ failure
IVDA	intravenous drug abuse	MPNST	malignant peripheral nerve sheath tumor
IVH	intraventricular hemorrhage	MPS	mucopolysaccharides
		MRA	magnetic resonance angiography
		MRI	magnetic resonance imaging
		MS	multiple sclerosis
		MSH	melanocyte-stimulating hormone
		MXT	methotrexate

J

JPA   juvenile pilocytic astrocytoma

K

KF   Kayser-Fleischer (rings)

L

LDH   lactate dehydrogenase
LE   lower extremity; lupus erythematosus
LFT   liver function test
LGB   lateral geniculate body
LH   luteinizing hormone
LHRH   luteinizing hormone-releasing hormone
LMN   lower motor neuron
LOAF   lumbricals 1 and 2, opponens pollicis, and abductor and flexor pollicis brevis

M

MBP   myelin basic protein
MCA   middle cerebral artery
MCP   metacarpophalangeal
MD   muscular dystrophy
MELAS   myopathy, encephalopathy, lactic acidosis, and strokes
MEN   multiple endocrine neoplasia

N

NAC   *N*-acetylcysteine
NAPA   *N*-acetylprocainamide
NCV   nerve conduction velocity
NE   norepinephrine
NF   neurofibromatosis
NIDDM   non-insulin-dependent diabetes mellitus
NMDA   *N*-methyl-D-aspartate
NMJ   neuromuscular junction
NSAID   nonsteroidal anti-inflammatory drug

O

OCP   oral contraceptive pill
OPLL   ossified posterior longitudinal ligament

P

PAM   L-phenylalanine mustard (melphalan)
PAS   periodic acid–Schiff
PCA   posterior cerebral artery

PCOM	posterior communicating artery
PCR	polymerase chain reaction
PCV	procarbazine, CCNU (lomustine), vincristine
PICA	posterior inferior cerebellar artery
PIF	prolactin-inhibiting hormone
PKU	phenylketonuria
PLL	posterior longitudinal ligament
PML	progressive multifocal leukoencephalopathy
PMN	polymorphonuclear neutrophils
PNET	primitive neuroectodermal tumor
PNS	peripheral nervous system
PPD	purified protein derivative
PR	prolactin
PSA	prostate specific antigen
PT	prothrombin time
PTH	parathyroid hormone
PTT	partial thromboplastin time
PVR	peripheral vascular resistance
PXA	pleomorphic xanthoastrocytoma

R

RA	rheumatoid arthritis
RBC	red blood cell
REM	rapid eye movement
REZ	root entry zone
RIND	reversible ischemic neurologic deficit
ROW	Rendu-Osler-Weber syndrome
RSD	reflex sympathetic dystrophy

S

SAH	subarachnoid hemorrhage
SBE	subacute bacterial endocarditis
SCA	superior cerebellar artery
SDH	subdural hematoma
SI	substantia innominata; sacroiliac
SIADH	syndrome of inappropriate antidiuretic hormone (secretion)

SLE	systemic lupus erythematosus
SMA	spinal muscle atrophy
SN	substantia nigra
SNpc	substantia nigra pars compacta
SNpr	substantia nigra pars reticulata
SSEP	somatosensory evoked potential
SSPE	subacute sclerosing panencephalitis
ST	subthalamus
SVR	systemic vascular resistance

T

T_3	triiodothyronine
T_4	thyroxine
TB	tuberculosis
TIA	transient ischemic attack
TNF	tumor necrosis factor
TORCH	toxoplasmosis, rubella, cytomegalovirus, and herpes simplex
tPA	tissue plasminogen activator
TRH	thyroid-releasing hormone
TS	tuberous sclerosis
TSH	thyroid-stimulating hormone

U

UBO	unidentified bright object
UMN	upper motor neuron

V

VA	ventroanterior; visceral afferent
VHL	Von Hippel-Lindau disease
VL	ventrolateral
VPI	ventral posterior inferior
VPL	ventroposterolateral
VPM	ventroposteromedial
vWF	von Willebrand's factor

W

WBC	white blood cell

Figure Acknowledgments

(Thieme books from which figures have been reproduced in this publication)

Figure 8 *Principles and Practice of Pediatric Neurosurgery*. Albright AL, Pollack IF, Adelson PD (Eds.). New York, NY: Thieme, 1999. (Figure 8-6)

Figure 14 *Teaching Atlas of Spine Imaging*. Ramsey RG. New York, NY: Thieme, 1999. (Page 86)

Figure 63 *Imaging of the Head and Neck*. Valvassori GE, Mafee MF, Carter BL. New York, NY: Thieme, 1995. (Figure 13.24)

Figure 67 *Microneurosurgery IV A*. Yasargil MG. New York, NY: Thieme, 1994. (Case 2.6 A,B)

Figure 74 *Principles and Practice of Pediatric Neurosurgery*. Albright AL, Pollack IF, Adelson PD (Eds.). New York, NY: Thieme, 1999. (Figures 25-6A-C)

Figure 77 *Principles and Practice of Pediatric Neurosurgery*. Albright AL, Pollack IF, Adelson PD (Eds.). New York, NY: Thieme, 1999. (Figures 25-6E,F)

Figure 92 *Cerebral Angiography, 2nd Edition*. Huber P, Krayenbühl H, Yasargil MG. New York, NY: Thieme, 1982. (Figure 546A)

Figure 111 *Principles and Practice of Pediatric Neurosurgery*. Albright AL, Pollack IF, Adelson PD (Eds.). New York, NY: Thieme, 1999. (Figure 31-2)

Figure 123 *Microneurosurgery IV B*. Yasargil MG. New York, NY: Thieme, 1996. (Figures 11.3A-C)

Figure 125 *Microneurosurgery IV B*. Yasargil MG. New York, NY: Thieme, 1996. (Figures 11.4 A,B)

Figure 128 *Cranial Microsurgery*. Sekhar LN, de Oliveira E. New York, NY: Thieme, 1998. (Figure 11.1)

Figure 131 *Neurosurgery Board Review*. Alleyne Jr. CH. New York, NY: Thieme, 1997. (Figure 34)

Figure 157 *Differential Diagnosis in Head and Neck Imaging*. Vogl TJ, Balzer J, Mack M, Steger S. New York, NY: Thieme, 1999. (Figures 3.13B,C)

Figure 159 *Neurosurgery Board Review*. Alleyne Jr. CH. New York, NY: Thieme, 1997. (Figure 1)

Figure 162 *Principles and Practice of Pediatric Neurosurgery*. Albright AL, Pollack IF, Adelson PD (Eds.). New York, NY: Thieme, 1999. (Figures 11-5A,B)

Figure 165 *Neurosurgery Board Review*. Alleyne Jr. CH. New York, NY: Thieme, 1997. (Figure 6)

Figure 166 *Neurosurgery Board Review*. Alleyne Jr. CH. New York, NY: Thieme, 1997. (Figure 2)

Figure 167 *Neurosurgery Board Review*. Alleyne Jr. CH. New York, NY: Thieme, 1997. (Figure 5)

Figure 169 *Neurosurgery Board Review*. Alleyne Jr. CH. New York, NY: Thieme, 1997. (Figure 4)

Figure 171 *Imaging of the Head and Neck*. Valvassori GE, Mafee MF, Carter BL. New York, NY: Thieme, 1995. (Figures 13.62A,B)

Figure 174 *Principles and Practice of Pediatric Neurosurgery*. Albright AL, Pollack IF, Adelson PD (Eds.). New York, NY: Thieme, 1999. (Figure 2-5)

Figures 179A,B *Teaching Atlas of Spine Imaging*. Ramsey RG. New York, NY: Thieme, 1999. (Pages 599-600, Figures A and C)

Figure 182 *Neurosurgery Board Review*. Alleyne Jr. CH. New York, NY: Thieme, 1997. (Figure 18)

Figure 190 *Neurosurgery Board Review*. Alleyne Jr. CH. New York, NY: Thieme, 1997. (Figure 26)

Figure 205 *Cranial Microsurgery*. Sekhar LN, de Oliveira E. New York, NY: Thieme, 1998. (Figures 20-14A,B)

Figure 220   *Cranial Microsurgery.* Sekhar LN, de Oliveira E. New York, NY: Thieme, 1998. (Figures 40-104A,E)

Figure 254   *Teaching Atlas of Spine Imaging.* Ramsey RG. New York, NY: Thieme, 1999. (Page 93)

Figure 256   *Neurosurgery Board Review.* Alleyne Jr. CH. New York, NY: Thieme, 1997. (Figure 16)

Figure 258   *Principles and Practice of Pediatric Neurosurgery.* Albright AL, Pollack IF, Adelson PD (Eds.). New York, NY: Thieme, 1999. (Figure 39-10)

Figures 269A-C   *Teaching Atlas of Spine Imaging.* Ramsey RG. New York, NY: Thieme, 1999. (Pages 611-612, Figures C,E,H)

Figure 270   *Teaching Atlas of Spine Imaging.* Ramsey RG. New York, NY: Thieme, 1999. (Page 834)

Figure 275   *Neurosurgery Board Review.* Alleyne Jr. CH. New York, NY: Thieme, 1997. (Figure 32)

Figure 280   *Neurosurgery Board Review.* Alleyne Jr. CH. New York, NY: Thieme, 1997. (Figure 31)

Figure 283   *Neurosurgery Board Review.* Alleyne Jr. CH. New York, NY: Thieme, 1997. (Figure 19)

Figures 293A,B   *Teaching Atlas of Spine Imaging.* Ramsey RG. New York, NY: Thieme, 1999. (Pages 739-740)

Figure 299   *Principles and Practice of Pediatric Neurosurgery.* Albright AL, Pollack IF, Adelson PD (Eds.). New York, NY: Thieme, 1999. (Figure 19-11A)

Figure 309   *Neurosurgery Board Review.* Alleyne Jr. CH. New York, NY: Thieme, 1997. (Figure 25)

Figure 310   *Imaging of the Head and Neck.* Valvassori GE, Mafee MF, Carter BL. New York, NY: Thieme, 1995. (Figure 13.45)

Index